PERIODONTAL-RESTORATIVE INTERRELATIONSHIPS

ENSURING CLINICAL SUCCESS

PERIODONTAL-RESTORATIVE INTERRELATIONSHIPS
ENSURING CLINICAL SUCCESS

Paul A. Fugazzotto, DDS

Contributions by Frederick Hains, DDS,
and Sergio DePaoli, MD, DDS

⟨W⟩WILEY-BLACKWELL

A John Wiley & Sons, Inc., Publication

This edition first published 2011 © 2011 by John Wiley & Sons, Inc.

Wiley-Blackwell is an imprint of John Wiley & Sons, formed by the merger of Wiley's global Scientific, Technical and Medical business with Blackwell Publishing.

Registered office: John Wiley & Sons Ltd, The Atrium, Southern Gate, Chichester, West Sussex, PO19 8SQ, UK

Editorial offices: 2121 State Avenue, Ames, Iowa 50014-8300, USA
The Atrium, Southern Gate, Chichester, West Sussex, PO19 8SQ, UK
9600 Garsington Road, Oxford, OX4 2DQ, UK

For details of our global editorial offices, for customer services and for information about how to apply for permission to reuse the copyright material in this book please see our website at www.wiley.com/wiley-blackwell.

Library of Congress Cataloging-in-Publication Data

Fugazzotto, Paul A.
  Periodontal-restorative interrelationships : ensuring clinical success / Paul A. Fugazzotto.
      p.; cm.
  Includes bibliographical references and index.
  ISBN 978-0-8138-1167-3 (hardcover : alk. paper)
1. Periodontal disease–Treatment.   2. Dentistry, Operative.
I. Title.
  [DNLM: 1. Periodontal Diseases–surgery.   2. Dental Restoration, Permanent–methods.   3. Oral Surgical Procedures–methods.   4. Orthodontics, Corrective–methods. WU 240]
  RK361.F84 2011
  617.6′32–dc22
                                                    2010049402

A catalogue record for this book is available from the British Library.

This book is published in the following electronic formats: ePDF 9780470959664; ePub 9780470959671

Set in 10.5 on 12pt ITC Slimbach by
Toppan Best-set Premedia Limited
Printed and bound in Singapore by Markono Print Media Pte Ltd

2 2014

To my daughters Martina and Lara, and in memory of my son, Dante, the three stars in my universe.

Contents

Contributors

Editor/Author:

Paul A. Fugazzotto, DDS
Private Practice
Milton, MA, USA

Contributing Authors:

Frederick Hains, DDS
Fellow of the Academy of General Dentistry
Associate Clinical Professor
Department of General Dentistry
Boston University, Henry M. Goldman School of
Dental Medicine
Boston, MA, USA

Sergio DePaoli, MD, DDS
Clinical Instructor
University of Ancona
Private Practice
Ancona, Italy

Diagrams by Martina Fugazzotto

PERIODONTAL-RESTORATIVE INTERRELATIONSHIPS
ENSURING CLINICAL SUCCESS

Chapter 1
Examination and Diagnosis

Paul Fugazzotto and Sergio DePaoli

The periodontal prerequisites for maximization of long-term oral health are well established. Effective home-care efforts, maintainable probing depths (defined as 3 mm or less), no evidence of furcation involvements, and adequate bands of attached keratinized tissue to provide a stable fiber barrier in various clinical scenaria are well-accepted periodontal endpoints of therapy. Combined with appropriate management of carious and endodontic lesions, replacement of missing teeth, control of parafunctional habits, and establishment of a healthy, stable occlusion, such a periodontal milieu will help ensure maximization of patient comfort, function, and aesthetics in both the short and long terms.

It has become popular to speak of paradigm shifts in clinical dentistry. However, these shifts represent nothing more than alterations in the treatment approaches utilized to attain the aforementioned therapeutic goals. In addition, efforts must be made to utilize the least-involved and least-expensive therapies possible for ensuring these treatment outcomes.

Maximizing oral health and ameliorating patient concerns remain essential to ethical practice. When considering the utilization of various treatment approaches, it is important to listen to patient desires, determine patient needs, and ensure that the therapy to be employed is truly in the best interest of the patient. A thorough understanding of the predictability of appropriately performed therapies around natural teeth is crucial to the formulation of an ideal treatment plan for a given patient. This treatment plan is based upon a precise diagnosis of the patient's condition and recognition of all contributing etiologies. Such a diagnosis takes into consideration the patient's overall health and the entire dentition, treating each site as both an individual entity and as a component of the masticatory unit.

Establishment of such oral health is dependent upon first carrying out a thorough examination, so as to establish a comprehensive diagnosis of patient etiologies, needs, and required therapies.

Establishing an Appropriate Treatment Plan

A high-quality full series of radiographs must be taken. All full series of radiographs must employ two film/sensor sizes: a #2 film/sensor in posterior regions and a #1 film/sensor in anterior areas. Attempts at utilizing either a #1- or #2-size film/sensor in all areas of the mouth will result in an inability to properly position the film/sensor in the anterior regions, and lead to poorly angulated, nondiagnostic radiographs. Digital radiographs are preferable, due to the ability to manipulate the images and thus gain additional information, and the lesser radiation exposure to the patient. When necessary, three-dimensional images are utilized. Panorex films are not used, since their accuracy is not sufficient for providing useful information for constructing a comprehensive diagnosis.

The components of a thorough clinical examination include periodontal probing depths, assessment of clinical attachment levels, hard- and soft-tissue examination, models, and face-bow records. However, it is important to realize that a thorough examination begins with an open discussion with the individual patient, as a step in determining the patient's needs and desires. In this way, treatment plans may be formulated that are in the best interest of the patient and represent a greater value for the patient.

Prior to formulating a comprehensive treatment plan, all potential etiologies must be

Periodontal Restorative Interrelationships: Ensuring Clinical Success, First Edition. Edited by Paul A. Fugazzotto.
© 2011 by John Wiley & Sons, Inc. Published 2011 by John Wiley & Sons, Inc.

identified and assessed. In addition to systemic factors, these etiologies include, but are not limited to, periodontal disease, parafunction, caries, endodontic lesions, and trauma.

The treating clinician should always formulate an "ideal" treatment plan and present it to every patient. Appropriate and predictable treatment alternatives must be offered to the patient as well, to allow the patient to choose the treatment option to which he or she is best suited physically, financially, and psychologically.

In many situations, initial therapies, such as plaque control instruction, debridement, caries control, and endodontic assessment, must be carried out prior to establishment of the final treatment options.

While it is true that clinicians who fail to incorporate regenerative and implant therapies into their treatment armamentaria are depriving their patients of predictable therapeutic possibilities that afford unique treatment outcomes in a variety of situations, other proven therapies should not be abandoned too quickly.

Teeth that can be predictably restored to health through reasonable means should be maintained, if their retention is advantageous to the final treatment plan. Clinicians who claim to be implantologists, performing only implant therapy while ignoring periodontal and other pathologies, do patients a disservice. Such clinicians include practitioners who either perform inadequate periodontal therapy to predictably halt the disease process, or remove teeth that could be treated through predictable periodontal techniques.

It is inconceivable that any clinician would see only patients who require implant therapy, and demonstrate periodontal, endodontic, restorative, and occlusal health around all remaining teeth that are not to be extracted. Such a clinical outlook is at the expense of ethical, comprehensive care, and must be avoided at all times.

Clinical presentations of different patients may appear similar, despite dramatic differences in etiology and individual patient needs. It is crucial that the conscientious clinician utilize all tools at his or her disposal to differentiate between various clinical entities.

It is also imperative that the periodontal restorative dynamic be understood in its complexity, and managed comprehensively, to maximize treatment endpoints. All periodontal therapies have restorative ramifications. Similarly, all restorative therapies have periodontal ramifications. One of the goals of the conscientious clinician must be to determine the relative influence of each discipline on the treatment considered in a given clinical scenario, and manage all aspects of this interrelationship appropriately.

Most if not all clinicians would agree that reconstructive therapy must be grounded in sound periodontal prosthetic principles. It is important to realize the same is true for a single restoration.

Periodontal procedures cannot be considered without understanding their far-reaching restorative ramifications. All therapies succeed or fail depending upon how periodontal and restorative concerns are managed, both individually and as interdependent entities.

The introduction by Amsterdam and Cohen (1) of the concept of periodontal prosthesis almost 50 years ago helped to define this interrelationship. While complex, state of the art therapies were presented and the results were documented over decades, such execution was not the greatest contribution the concepts of periodontal prosthesis have made to modern clinical practice. Rather, periodontal prosthesis afforded clinicians something even more important. A system was presented by which comprehensive record taking, diagnosis, and treatment planning could be carried out with specific treatment endpoints in mind, resulting in long-term therapeutic success. The advent of implant therapy has done nothing to change this concept. Comprehensive care mandates thorough examination and record taking, a multifactorial diagnosis, and interdisciplinary treatment planning to maximize therapeutic outcomes. Case types may be categorized as follows.

THE PERIODONTAL RESTORATIVE CASE

A patient presents with significant periodontal concerns, manifesting themselves as hard- and soft-tissue changes, deepening pocket depths, and inflammation. In these situations, restorative therapy may be required to help improve the outcomes of comprehensive periodontal treatment. Restorative therapy often includes splinting of mobile teeth, coverage of sensitive roots, and correction of occlusal abnormalities to improve periodontal prognoses.

It is important to realize that while less mobility is always desirable, increased mobility patterns should not be viewed as a contraindication to periodontal or restorative therapies of various complexities. Increased mobility, if it is not to such a degree as to result in either continued dysfunction or tooth extraction, will not negatively impact long-term prognosis to a significant degree. However, should fixed partial dentures be contemplated to replace a missing tooth or teeth, additional teeth may be required to serve as abutments in the presence of increased tooth mobility, to afford the necessary stability to the fixed partial denture under function. Increasing mobility should be viewed as a highly significant negative factor when determining expected prognoses for various therapies, and may be an absolute contraindication, to performing complex treatments on given teeth rather than removing these teeth and replacing them with implant-supported prosthetics. This type of case will not be discussed in detail, as it is not the purpose of this text.

THE RESTORATIVE PERIODONTAL CASE

Maximization of long-term restorative treatment outcomes is highly dependent upon the periodontal milieu into which restorative therapy is placed. A harmonious occlusion, probing depths of 3 mm or less, no horizontal furcation involvements, stable bands of attached keratinized tissue of at least 3 mm in the apico-occlusal dimension and 2 mm in the buccolingual dimension, and restorative margin positions that are accessible to the patient for predictable home-care efforts are all prerequisites for attainment of successful restorative treatment outcomes.

The methods available to attain these goals will be discussed in detail throughout the text. A restorative periodontal case is one that requires periodontal intervention not to eliminate active periodontal diseases, but rather to appropriately prepare the periodontium for reception of restorative dentistry. Such therapies may include, for example, hard- and/or soft-tissue crown lengthening, soft-tissue augmentation, ondontoplasty, and frenectomy.

INTRODUCTION OF ORTHODONTIC THERAPY INTO EITHER CASE TYPE

Although this is not the format in which to discuss complex full-mouth orthodontic therapy, appropri-

ate utilization of orthodontic treatment approaches in isolated areas will significantly enhance the functional and aesthetic outcomes of therapy in both periodontal restorative cases and restorative periodontal cases. Such orthodontic utilization includes:

- alignment of malpositioned teeth to improve ease of patient home care
- alignment of malpositioned teeth to ameliorate off-angle functional and parafunctional forces
- establishment of more ideal occlusal planes
- establishment of flatter occlusal planes with shallower incisal guidance to help ameliorate forces being placed upon the anterior teeth
- tooth reangulation for ease of prosthetic therapy
- tooth reangulation to assist in patient home-care efforts
- tooth uprighting to help eliminate cemento-enamel junction position induced osseous defects (Figs. 1.1–1.6)
- tooth supereruption in anticipation of crown-lengthening osseous surgery in the aesthetic zone, to allow appropriate restoration and maintenance of a compromised tooth without negatively affecting patient aesthetics and/or allow crown lengthening without compromising the support of the adjacent teeth (Figs. 1.7–1.15)

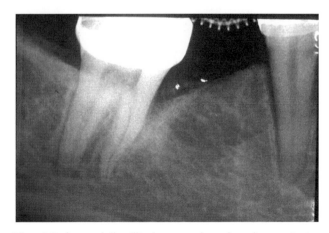

Fig. 1.1 A mesially tilted second molar demonstrates an infrabony defect due to cementoenamel junction positions.

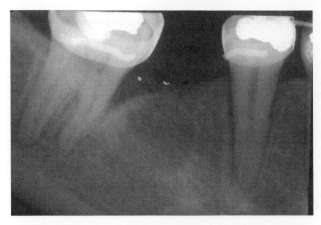

Fig. 1.2 Orthodontic uprighting of the tilted molar is beginning to eliminate the infrabony defect that was present.

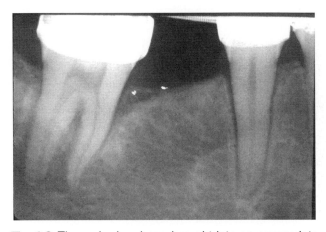

Fig. 1.3 The molar has been brought into an appropriate position. No infrabony defect remains. Note the "bone regeneration" on the mesial aspect of the molar.

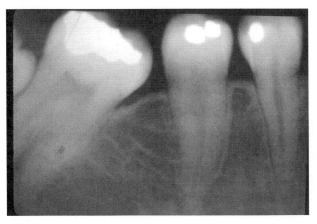

Fig. 1.4 A severely tilted second molar demonstrates an "infrabony defect" on its mesial aspect. Note the positions of the cementoenamel junctions.

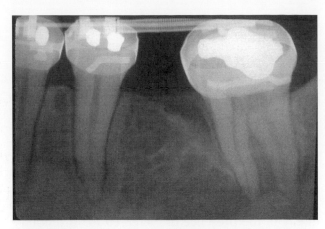

Fig. 1.5 Molar uprighting is proceeding. Note the elimination of the defect on the mesial aspect of the molar.

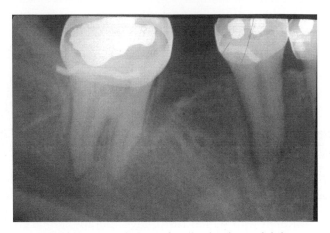

Fig. 1.6 Upon completion of orthodontic uprighting, no infrabony defect remains on the mesial aspect of the second molar.

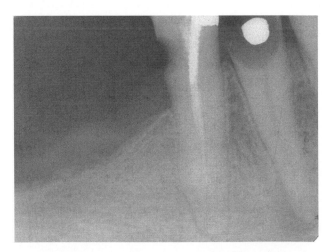

Fig. 1.7 A 51-year-old female presents with caries on her mandibular right first and second premolars. The caries on the first premolar extends approximately 3 mm apical to the alveolar crest. Attempts at crown-lengthening osseous surgery around the first premolar would require removal of extensive supporting bone from the adjacent teeth.

6

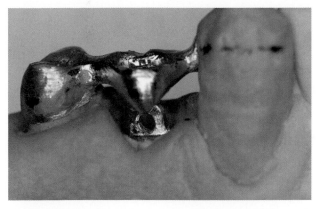

Fig. 1.8 A laboratory view of the fixed orthodontic appliance that will be cemented in place and will engage the root of the mandibular first premolar.

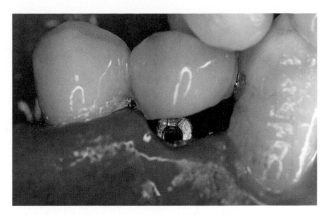

Fig. 1.11 A buccal view of the supereruptive appliance and temporary prosthesis in place.

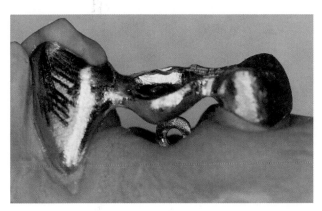

Fig. 1.9 A lingual view of the fabricated orthodontic appliance.

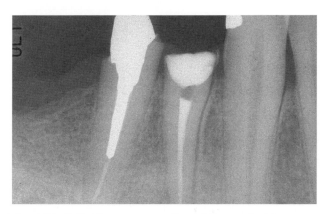

Fig. 1.12 Following supereruption of the root of the mandibular first premolar, crown-lengthening osseous surgery may now be performed without unduly compromising the alveolar support of the adjacent teeth.

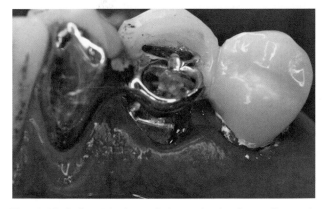

Fig. 1.10 A lingual view of the orthodontic appliance in place. The area is temporized around the appliance to help ameliorate the patient's aesthetic concerns.

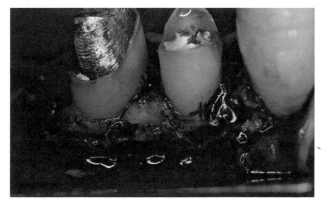

Fig. 1.13 Crown-lengthening osseous surgery has been performed around both mandibular premolars.

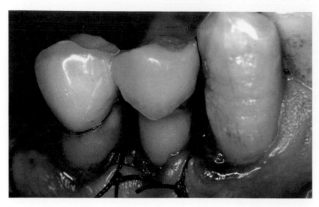

Fig. 1.14 Following suturing of the mucoperiosteal flaps at alveolar crest and replacement of the provisional restoration, the extent of crown lengthening that has been attained is evident.

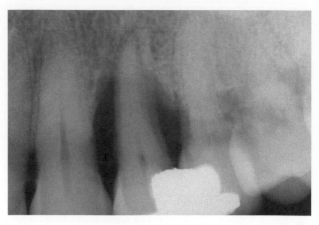

Fig. 1.16 A 62-year-old male presents with a hopeless prognosis for his maxillary left first premolar. Note the extensive bone loss around this tooth, which is affecting the support of the adjacent teeth.

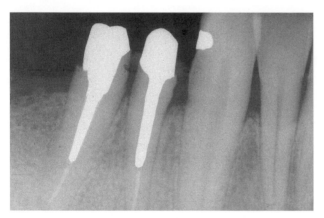

Fig. 1.15 A radiograph taken after post and core fabrication and insertion into the mandibular premolars demonstrates the relationship of the planned restorative margins to the alveolar crests.

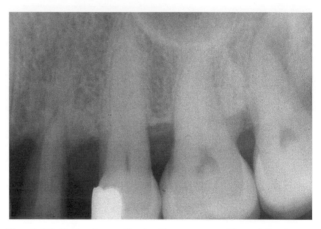

Fig. 1.17 Following orthodontic supereruption of the hopeless maxillary left first premolar, the osseous defects that were present have been resolved, with no loss of alveolar bone on the facing surfaces of the adjacent teeth. The patient now presents with an ideal alveolar crest for implant placement, and maximization of the periodontal health of the adjacent teeth.

- supereruption prior to tooth extraction to extrude hard and soft tissues, improve aesthetics in the papillary and/or marginal areas, and afford site preparation in anticipation of either pontic or implant crown placement (Figs. 1.16–1.20)

CLINICAL EXAMPLE ONE

A 51-year-old female presents with extensive caries on her mandibular right first and second premolars. The caries on the first premolar extends approximately 3 mm apical to the osseous crest. Attempts at crown-lengthening osseous surgery would result in removal of extensive and significant supporting alveolar bone from the distal aspect of the cuspid and the mesial aspect of the second premolar (Fig. 1.7).

Following caries excavation on both mandibular premolars, an impression is taken and a fixed orthodontic appliance is fabricated, which will be utilized to supererupt the root of the first premolar. This orthodontic appliance will be fixed to the cuspid and second premolar, and will engage a

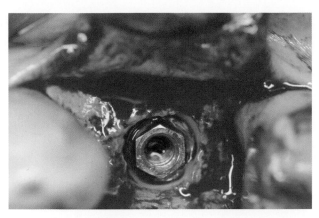

Fig. 1.18 The alveolar bone crest, which has been repositioned through orthodontic supereruption, is evident following implant placement in the maxillary left first premolar position.

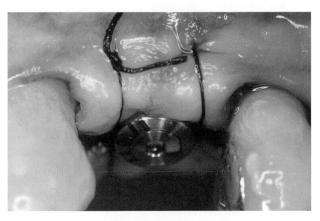

Fig. 1.19 The mucoperiosteal flaps are sutured in the desired positions with interrupted silk sutures.

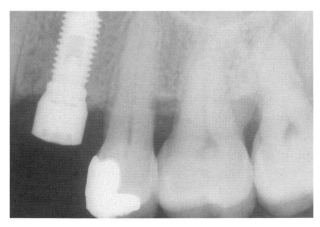

Fig. 1.20 A radiograph taken after implant placement demonstrates the ideal contour and position of the alveolar crest, which was rebuilt utilizing orthodontic supereruptive techniques.

specifically designed post in the root of the first premolar (Figs. 1.8, 1.9). Once the orthodontic appliance is inserted, a temporary provisional restoration is placed over both the first and second premolars to help satisfy the patient's aesthetic concerns (Figs. 1.10, 1.11). Following supereruption of the root of the first premolar, the orthodontic appliance and the orthodontic post in the root of the first premolar are removed. A radiograph taken at this time demonstrates that the supererupted mandibular first premolar can now be safely crown lengthened without compromising the prognoses of the adjacent teeth (Fig. 1.12).

Crown-lengthening osseous surgery is carried out (Fig. 1.13). The technical aspects of this therapy will be described in detail in Chapter 2. Following suturing of the buccal and lingual mucoperiosteal flaps at osseous crest with interrupted silk sutures, the provisional restorations are replaced on the crown-lengthened first and second mandibular premolars (Fig. 1.14). The extent of crown lengthening that has been attained is evident. A radiograph taken following post and core buildup and preparation of the mandibular right first and second premolars demonstrates that adequate dimensions are present between the planned restorative margins and the osseous crest to allow development of a healthy periodontal attachment apparatus. Neither the cuspid nor second premolar have been compromised by the crown-lengthening therapy that has been carried out (Fig. 1.15).

CLINICAL EXAMPLE TWO

A 62-year-old patient presents with a periodontally hopeless maxillary left first premolar. Radiographically, extensive osseous loss is present around this tooth. In addition, the thin nature of the remaining supporting alveolar bone on the distal aspect of the maxillary cuspid and the mesial aspect of the maxillary second premolar is evident (Fig. 1.16). Extraction of the first premolar and performance of simultaneous regenerative therapy, with or without implant placement, would place this thin supporting alveolar bone at risk, and potentially compromise the long-term prognoses of the cuspid and second premolar.

Following orthodontic supereruption of the hopeless root of the first premolar, both resolution of the aforementioned periodontal defect and maintenance of all supporting bone on the adjacent teeth are evident (Fig. 1.17). This root may now be extracted and an implant safely placed, without compromising the prognoses of the adjacent teeth.

Following reflection of buccal and palatal mucoperiosteal flaps, an implant is placed in the position of the maxillary left first premolar (Fig. 1.18). The interproximal alveolar bone, which has been maintained and rebuilt through orthodontic supereruption, is evident. The mucoperiosteal flaps are sutured at the desired positions, utilizing interrupted 4-0 silk sutures (Fig. 1.19). A radiograph taken following implant placement demonstrates an ideal alveolar ridge form and the health of the periodontal attachment apparatus on the facing surfaces of the adjacent teeth (Fig. 1.20).

CLINICAL EXAMPLE THREE

A 47-year-old female presents with a fractured maxillary central incisor (Fig. 1.21). A radiograph demonstrates extensive bone loss between the fractured maxillary central incisor and the adjacent lateral incisor (Fig. 1.22). Extraction of this tooth, with or without concomitant regenerative therapy and/or implant placement, would result in significant shrinkage of the soft tissues and loss of the interdental papilla in the region.

Following removal of the fractured portion of the central incisor, the root is supererupted with a fixed orthodontic appliance (Fig. 1.23). A radiograph taken during the supereruptive process demonstrates how the attachment apparatus and alveolar bone have been "brought coronally" along with the retained root of the maxillary central

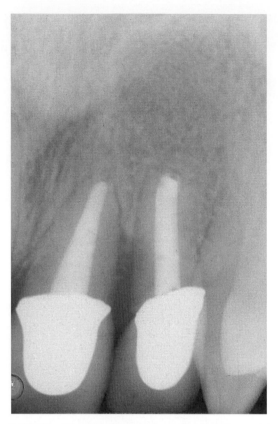

Fig. 1.22 Significant bone loss is evident radiographically between the fractured central incisor and the adjacent lateral incisor.

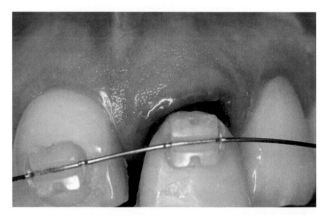

Fig. 1.23 Following removal of the fractured portion of the central incisor, the retained root is supererupted utilizing a fixed orthodontic appliance.

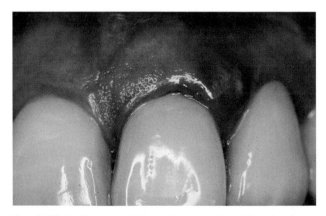

Fig. 1.21 A 47-year-old female presents with a fractured maxillary central incisor.

incisor (Fig. 1.24). The retained root is extracted without reflecting a flap, so as to minimize trauma to the hard and soft tissues in the area (Fig. 1.25). Examination of the extracted root

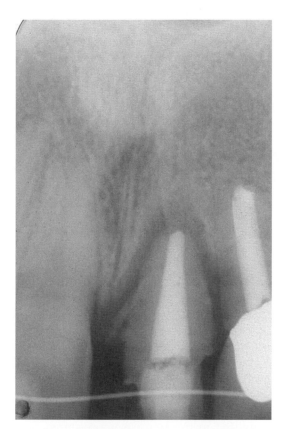

Fig. 1.24 A radiograph taken during the supereruptive process demonstrates coronal repositioning of the alveolar bone between the central and lateral incisors.

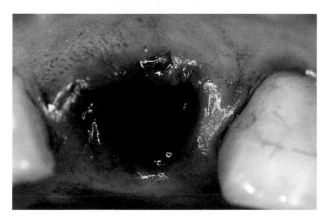

Fig. 1.25 The retained root of the central incisor is removed without reflecting a mucoperiosteal flap, so as to minimize trauma to the hard and soft tissues in the area.

demonstrates the orientation of the periodontal ligament fibers, which results during supereruption (Fig. 1.26). The attachment of these fibers to the surrounding alveolar bone is critical when this bone is to be repositioned coronally.

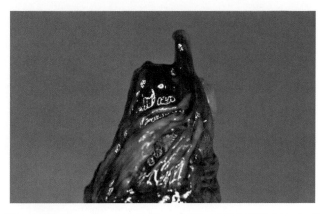

Fig. 1.26 Note the orientation of the periodontal ligament fibers on the root surface, as a result of the supereruptive process.

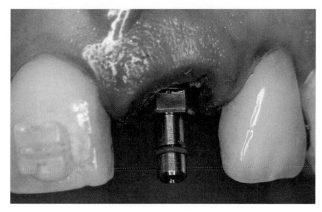

Fig. 1.27 Following implant placement, the soft-tissue papillae have been maintained.

Following implant placement, retention of the interproximal soft-tissue papillae is evident (Fig. 1.27). The volume of bone that has been brought into position on the mesial aspect of the lateral incisor is highlighted in a radiograph taken following implant placement (Fig. 1.28). This alveolar bone will be crucial to the support and maintenance of the interproximal papilla, and thus the patient's aesthetics following completion of therapy. Retention of the interproximal papillae and acceptable aesthetics are noted following temporization of the implant (Fig. 1.29).

While supereruption offers considerable potential clinical advantages, it is imperative that the possible disadvantages of such therapy be recognized and considered when formulating a comprehensive treatment plan. These disadvantages

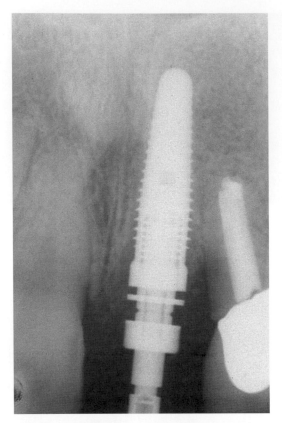

Fig. 1.28 A radiograph taken following implant placement demonstrates the extensive repositioning of the alveolar bone which has taken place on the mesial aspect of the lateral incisor. This bone will be crucial to the support and maintenance of the interproximal soft-tissue papilla.

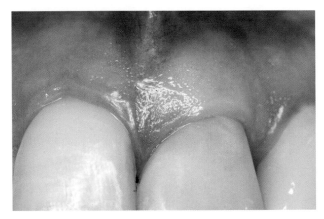

Fig. 1.29 Following implant temporization, retention of the interproximal papilla between the implant and the lateral incisor is evident.

include the time and expense involved in super-eruption. In addition, supererupting a maxillary lateral incisor to the point where it will demonstrate a poor crown-to-root ratio following restoration is not in a patient's best interest. Orthodontic considerations will be discussed in Chapter 6.

INTRODUCTION OF REGENERATIVE AND/OR IMPLANT THERAPIES

Such treatments may impact the partially edentulous patient on a number of levels, including replacement of less-predictable therapies, replacement of more costly therapies, augmentation of existing therapies, introduction of newer therapies, and simplification of therapy. Use of implants is not the topic under consideration in this text. For a detailed discussion, see Fugazzotto (2009) (2).

Regardless of which therapeutic approaches are utilized, maximization of treatment outcomes is dependent upon identification of etiologic factors, a thorough and insightful diagnosis, and formulation of a multidisciplinary, comprehensive treatment plan. The importance of these considerations is highlighted in the two cases presented below.

CLINICAL EXAMPLE FOUR

A 57-year-old male, presented with severe wear of his maxillary and mandibular anterior teeth, caries on many older restorations, and general aesthetic dissatisfaction (Figs. 1.30, 1.31). Prior to formulating a treatment plan and initiating active therapy, a determination must be made as to whether or not this is an example of tooth wear and loss of vertical dimension, or if vertical dimension has been maintained as the anterior teeth have worn due to the presence of a parafunctional habit. Examination of the occlusal surfaces of the maxillary and mandibular posterior teeth (Figs. 1.32, 1.33) demonstrates retention of the anatomy initially developed in the restorations and a lack of occlusal wear. Loss of vertical dimension has not occurred.

The severe anterior wear that has been noted is a result of the patient bringing his lower jaw into a protrusive position and demonstrating a parafunctional habit solely on his anterior teeth. As these teeth have worn down, the maxillary anterior teeth have supererupted. As a result,

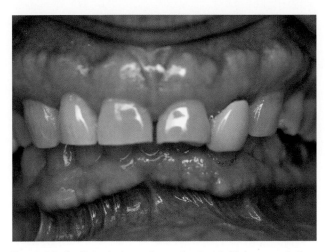

Fig. 1.30 A clinical view of a patient at initial presentation. Note the severe wear of the maxillary and mandibular anterior teeth.

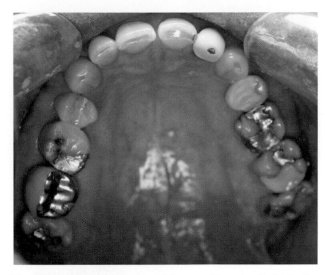

Fig. 1.32 An occlusal view of the maxillary teeth. Note the lack of occlusal wear.

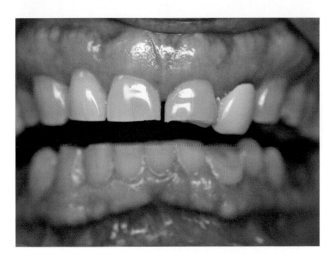

Fig. 1.31 Severe wear of the mandibular left cuspid by the opposing full coverage restoration is evident.

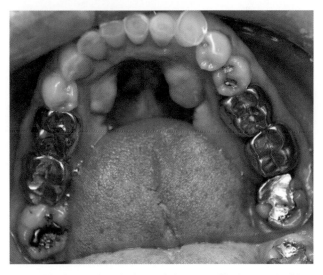

Fig. 1.33 An occlusal view of the mandibular teeth. Note the lack of occlusal wear.

crown-lengthening osseous surgery and restoration of the teeth in question will be required to address the patient's aesthetics concerns.

Accurate full arch impressions were taken and diagnostic casts poured. A face-bow transfer was taken. The diagnostic casts were duplicated in the dental laboratory and all of the casts were cross mounted on an Artex Articulator (Jensen Industries, North Haven, CT). Diagnostic waxups were performed on the duplicate casts as follows: The casts were modified to reposition the gingival margins to ideal aesthetic levels. These levels were determined by measuring the full-coverage restoration

of the maxillary lateral incisor. As no wear had occurred to the occlusal surface of this restoration and the mesiodistal dimensions of the teeth were intact, the ideal lengths of the original teeth could be assessed utilizing well-established proportional measurements. Taking the existing maxillary anterior incisal positions as ideal, the casts were modified accordingly to provide the determined ideal tooth lengths (Fig. 1.34).

A vacuform shell was fabricated in the laboratory on a modified diagnostic cast, which

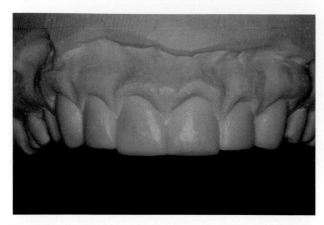

Fig. 1.34 The mounted models have been carved to attain the desired gingival margin positions, and a waxup of the models has been carried out.

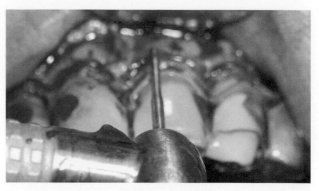

Fig. 1.36 Osseous resection has been carried out to ensure a 2.5-mm dimension between the osseous crest and the desired final gingival margin.

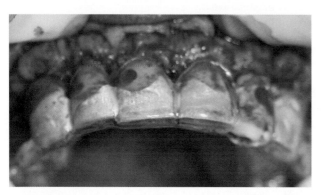

Fig. 1.35 The fabricated guide is placed on the maxillary teeth following flap reflection.

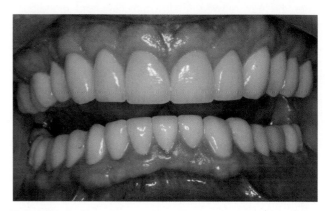

Fig. 1.37 A clinical view of the final restorations in place.

demarcated the desired gingival margin positions. Following full thickness flap reflection, the guide was placed over the maxillary teeth. Osseous resective therapy was performed to ensure a 2.5-mm dimension between the osseous crests and the demarcated gingival margin positions on the guide (Figs. 1.35, 1.36). It is crucial that this dimension be attained, to ensure development of the soft tissues at the appropriate levels following healing. It is also necessary to reduce buccal osseous ledging appropriately. As will be discussed in Chapter 2, failure to do so will result in the soft-tissue margins healing too far coronally, due to the soft tissues having to traverse the buccal osseous ledging and make their way to the tooth surfaces.

Following appropriate periodontal crown-lengthening surgery, with buccal and palatal/lingual reduction being carried out as necessary,

final full-coverage restorations were placed to restore the teeth following caries excavation and to address the patient's aesthetic desires (Fig. 1.37). Two bite appliances were fabricated. The patient wore the maxillary appliance at night, and the mandibular appliance during the day.

CLINICAL EXAMPLE FIVE

A 62-year-old male, presented with severe wear and chipping of his maxillary and mandibular anterior teeth (Figs. 1.38, 1.39). Extensive caries was noted around all abutments of the existing fixed prostheses. Teeth numbers 3, 7, and all remaining mandibular molars, demonstrated poor long-term prognoses due to a combination of caries and periodontal disease. A 15-mm long, 4.1-mm wide IMZ implant had been in place for over 15 years, and demonstrated no peri-implant bone loss, in the position of tooth number 18.

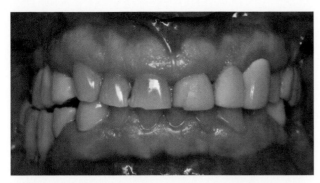

Fig. 1.38 A patient presented with worn and chipped maxillary and mandibular anterior teeth.

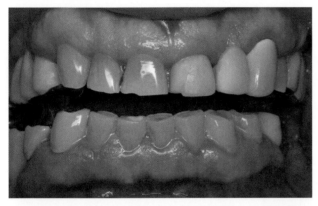

Fig. 1.39 The compromised condition of the maxillary and mandibular anterior teeth is evident.

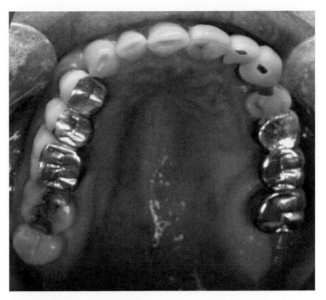

Fig. 1.40 An occlusal view of the maxillary arch demonstrates significant occlusal wear.

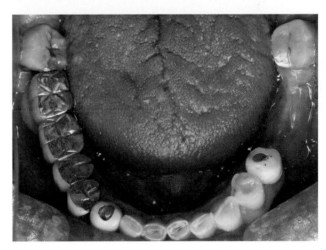

Fig. 1.41 An occlusal view of the mandibular arch demonstrates severe occlusal wear.

During the course of diagnosis, a determination had to be made whether this patient demonstrated loss of vertical dimension, or a situation similar to that of the previous patient (no loss of vertical dimension, but wear of the anterior teeth due to an eccentric parafunctional habit). Severe occlusal wear was noted upon examination of the occlusal surfaces of the maxillary and mandibular posterior teeth (Figs. 1.40, 1.41). As a result, it was determined that this patient had lost vertical dimension. Therefore, crown-lengthening osseous surgery was not required. Rather, an appropriate vertical dimension must be reestablished, and the teeth restored to this dimension.

The mounted diagnostic casts were next examined (Fig. 1.42). Because the mesiodistal dimensions of the maxillary anterior teeth had not changed as a result of tooth wear, a determination could be made as to the pretraumatic, ideal lengths of these teeth, utilizing well-established propor-

tions. Following such calculations, it was determined that the patient would have to have his vertical dimension increased by 5 mm in the anterior region (Fig. 1.43), to accommodate reestablishment of appropriate maxillary and mandibular tooth lengths, and acceptable overbite and overjet relationships.

However, a patient's vertical dimension cannot be increased by such an extent without first ensuring that these changes will not induce discomfort or other untoward symptoms. This

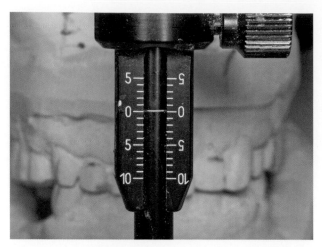

Fig. 1.42 Impressions were taken and the models were mounted with face-bow records.

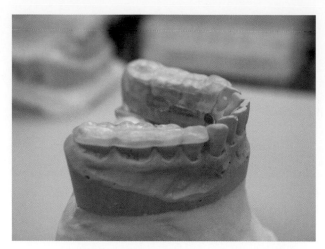

Fig. 1.44 A view of a mandibular occlusal repositioning appliance, which had been made for another patient.

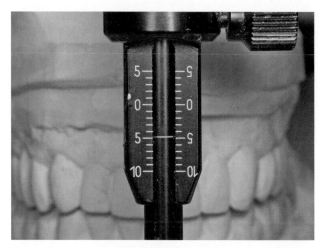

Fig. 1.43 The patient's vertical dimension was increased by 5 mm in the anterior region.

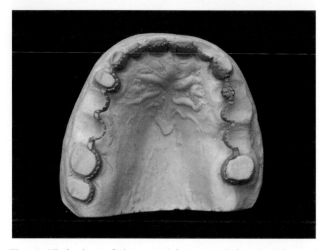

Fig. 1.45 A view of the metal framework for the planned maxillary provisional restoration.

determination must be made before fixed temporization is carried out. To accomplish this, a mandibular occlusal repositioning appliance (MORA) was fabricated and inserted. This appliance overlays the mandibular teeth, is worn at all times except during mastication, and is wholly reversible (Fig. 1.44). Such an appliance may also be used to help assess planned jaw repositioning. After 6 weeks of appliance use, the patient exhibited no untoward symptoms. It was therefore determined that he could be restored to the desired vertical dimension.

Because of the extensive regenerative and implant therapies required, treatment would last

approximately 18 months. This fact, combined with the need to establish a new vertical dimension for the patient, mandated the use of cast-metal-framework provisional restorations. Wire-reinforced provisional restorations are never utilized, due to their relative frailty. All too often wires serve no purpose other than to hold together broken portions of the provisional restorations. Rather, the provisional restorations are reinforced with the cast framework.

Because implants were to be placed following bone regeneration, and retrofitted to the existing prostheses following osseointegration, specific framework designs were employed (Figs. 1.45,

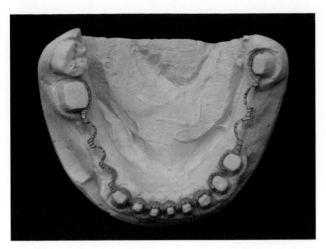

Fig. 1.46 A view of the metal framework for the planned mandibular provisional restoration.

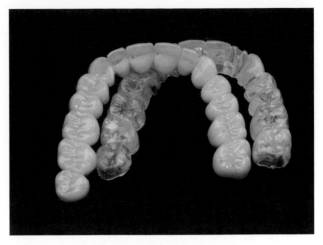

Fig. 1.47 A view of the metal framework reinforced maxillary provisional restoration, and the clear shell of the provisional restoration, which will be relined and will serve as a precise surgical guide.

1.46). The shape of this framework afforded the desired reinforcement of the provisional restoration, while allowing the pontic areas to be hollowed out, so that the provisional restoration could be retrofitted to the osseointegrated implants utilizing abutments and acrylic. Once the osseointegrated implants were incorporated into the provisional restorations, hopeless teeth that had been utilized to support the provisional restorations would be extracted. They would be replaced with implants at the time of tooth extraction with concomitant regenerative therapy, or following regenerative therapy in the extraction socket areas, depending upon the residual extraction socket morphologies and the ability to ideally position implants into the extraction sockets. The maxillary and mandibular full arch provisional restorations were fabricated (Figs. 1.47, 1.48), in the above-described manner.

Therapy proceeded as follows:

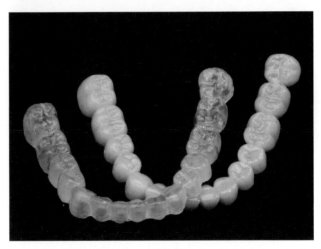

Fig. 1.48 A view of the mandibular metal framework reinforced provisional restoration, and the clear shell of the provisional restoration, which will be relined and will serve as a precise surgical guide.

A. The patient's maxillary and mandibular arches were provisionalized in one day (Fig. 1.49). The temporary fixed prostheses were then removed. At the time of provisional restoration fabrication, clear duplicate shell provisional restorations were fabricated. These clear provisional restorations were to be utilized as surgical guides during implant placement. To properly locate the guides during implant placement, the clear provisional restorations were relined with acrylic to the prepared teeth (Fig. 1.50). The pontic areas of planned implant placement had tubes placed into them. The pontics were then filled with acrylic, providing rigid guides for ideal implant placement. The metal frame provisional prostheses were then cemented.

B. The necessary mandibular posterior ridge augmentation therapy was carried out. During this visit, hopeless teeth numbers 3 and 7 were also extracted, and regenerative therapy was performed in the extraction socket areas.

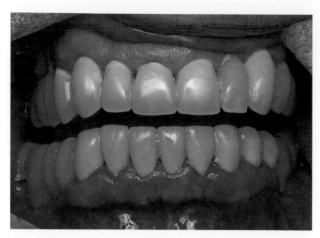

Fig. 1.49 The patient's maxillary and mandibular arches have been provisionalized during one clinical visit.

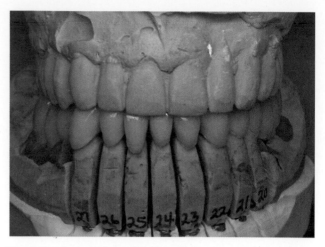

Fig. 1.51 A view of mandibular restorations on the implants and natural teeth on the models.

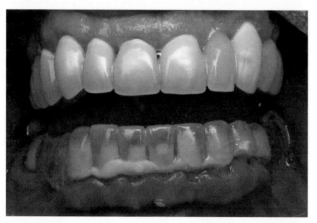

Fig. 1.50 Clear shells of the provisional restorations are relined and will serve as precise surgical guides.

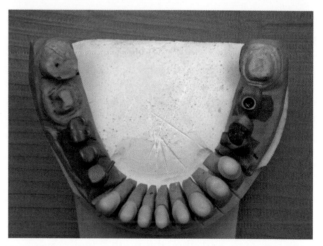

Fig. 1.52 A view of the metal frameworks on the implants and natural teeth in the mandibular arch.

C. Following maturation of the regenerating hard tissues, implants were placed in the desired maxillary and mandibular positions.

D. Upon completion of osseointegration, impressions were taken and fabrication of the final implant and natural-tooth-supported prostheses began (Fig. 1.51, 1.52).

E. The final restorations were completed and inserted in the patient's mouth (Fig. 1.53).

F. A bite appliance was fabricated to be worn at night indefinitely by the patient.

Disparate etiologies may result in clinical pictures that at first seem similar. However, appropriate patient examination and diagnosis will identify contributing etiologies and direct the formulation of an appropriate interdisciplinary,

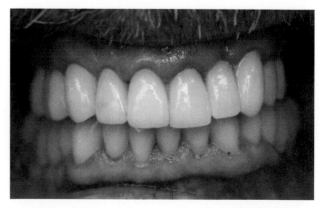

Fig. 1.53 A view of the maxillary and mandibular final restorations in place.

comprehensive treatment plan. Failure to perform such therapy significantly compromises long-term patient outcomes.

Determining Periodontal Treatment Endpoints

Effective patient home care, coupled with regular professional maintenance, are the cornerstones of all successful therapy. A patient who is unwilling or unable to demonstrate the necessary level of plaque removal efficacy and commitment should never be considered a candidate for interdisciplinary therapy. Rather, all efforts must be made through instructional, motivational, technical, and chemical means to help the patient in question control plaque levels and thus provide a reasonable milieu for the acceptance of the necessary dentistry. Failure to demand such a level of plaque control results in therapeutic failure, and increased levels of frustration and anxiety for both the patient and the treating clinicians.

While the patient has an obligation to make every effort to perform appropriate plaque control, it is imperative that the treating clinicians provide the patient with a milieu that is most conducive to effective plaque control, and that provides the greatest chance of a favorable long-term prognosis.

When faced with active periodontal disease, one of seven therapies may be employed (see Table 1.1).

1. *No treatment*: Whether such a decision is due to the patient's refusal of active therapy, or the patient's physical, financial, or psychological inability to undergo the necessary treatments, it is important to recognize the short- and long-term risks to oral and overall health represented by such a decision. Periodontal diseases are self-propagating disease entities. If no active therapy is carried out to halt disease progress, extension of the disease will result in tooth loss. When a patient refuses necessary care, every effort should be made to motivate the patient to pursue treatment, and to adapt the treatment to the individual patient.
2. *Subgingival debridement and institution of a regular professional prophylaxis schedule*: In many cases, such an approach does not halt the ongoing periodontal disease processes, but merely slows the rate of attachment loss. This treatment option is indicated for patients who are physically, financially, or psychologically unable to undergo more comprehensive therapy, in an attempt to delay tooth loss. Other than patients of an advanced age who have demonstrated moderate attachment loss, most patients are ill suited to such actuarial therapeutic regimens. The potential dangers to adjacent teeth must also be recognized.
3. *Surgical therapies aimed at defect debridement and/or pocket reduction*: These treatment approaches represent a significant compromise in therapy. As a patient who has undergone such surgical intervention is left with a milieu that is highly susceptible to further periodontal breakdown, the need for retreatment and the potential damage to the attachment apparatuses of adjacent teeth must be weighed. This treatment option offers minimal advantages over debridement, and no advantages when compared to the treatment approaches described below.
4. *Resective periodontal surgical therapy, including elimination of furcation involvements, in an effort to ensure a post therapeutic attachment apparatus characterized by a connective tissue attachment to the root surface, followed by a short junctional epithelial adhesion to the root surface, and elimination of probing depths greater than 3 mm*: While such a treatment approach offers the greatest chance of preventing reinitiation of periodontal disease processes, it must be utilized appropriately. Osseous resective therapy that results in irreversible compromise of a given tooth, the initiation of secondary occlusal trauma due to reduced periodontal support and a poor crown-to-root ratio, or an aesthetically unacceptable treatment result should not be considered ideal therapy, especially as the advent of regenerative and implant therapies affords additional treatment options in previously untenable scenarios.
5. *Periodontal regenerative therapy aimed at rebuilding lost attachment apparatus and surrounding alveolar bone*: Due to a history of misunderstanding of the indications and contraindications of periodontal regenerative therapy, and less than fully defined

Table 1.1. Treatment options for periodontally involved teeth.

Options	Advantages	Disadvantages
No treatment	Patient undergoes least amount of therapy.	Disease will continue to progress resulting in disease loss.
Subgingival debridement	Patient undergoes minimal amount of therapy. Ongoing disease process is slowed.	Disease process is not halted. Continued loss of attachment apparatus and eventual loss of teeth will occur.
Surgical debridement and/or pocket reduction	More thorough debridement than previous treatment options	Reinstitution of disease process is common. Attachment loss and eventual tooth loss
Resective periodontal therapy with elimination of furcations and no pocket depths greater than 3 mm	Delivers the most predictable attachment apparatus post therapy. Periodontal prognosis is optimized.	Patient must undergo various surgical therapies. Treatment is highly technique sensitive.
Regenerative therapy to rebuild lost attachment apparatus and alveolar bone	Lost tissues are regained. Prognosis is excellent when therapy is successful.	Poor understanding of prerequisites to delivery of therapy compromises results. Treatment is not as predictable as resective therapy.
Tooth removal with implant placement and regeneration if needed	Questionable teeth are eliminated. Therapy is predictable. Prognosis is excellent.	Teeth are lost. Highest cost of therapy
Combination of above therapies	As listed above	Potential highest cost of therapy

diagnostic systems, treatment outcomes have proven highly inconsistent. When utilized in the appropriate manner in stringently diagnosed and selected periodontal defects, guided tissue regeneration yields highly predictable treatment outcomes. The advent of new materials offers the potential for even more impressive regenerative results.

6. *Tooth removal with either simultaneous regenerative therapy and implant insertion or guided bone regeneration with subsequent implant placement and restoration:* Despite their high level of predictability, regenerative and implant therapies must not be viewed as a panacea. To remove teeth that may be predictably maintained through more conservative therapies that will yield acceptable treatment outcomes is unconscionable. It is also unreasonable to maintain compromised teeth that will eventually be lost or to subject a patient to an inordinate amount of therapy or expense to keep teeth that may be more simply and predictably replaced by implants.

7. *A combination of the above therapies:* Patients are all too often viewed as either "periodontal patients" or "implant patients." Patients are neither.

Rationale for Pocket-Elimination Periodontal Surgery

Pocket elimination, which has long been advanced as one of the primary endpoints of periodontal therapy, is most frequently accomplished through osseous resective surgery.

The primary goal of pocket-elimination therapy is to deliver to the patient an environment that is conducive to predictable, long-term periodontal health, both clinically and histologically. As such, the objectives are as follows:

1. Pocket elimination or reduction to such a level where thorough subgingival plaque control is predictable for both the patient and the practitioner.

2. A physiologic gingival contour that is conducive to plaque-control measures. Soft-tissue concavities, in the area of the interproximal col and elsewhere, soft-tissue clefts, and marked gingival margin discrepancies are eliminated.
3. The establishment of the most plaque-resistant attachment apparatus possible. This includes the elimination of long junctional epithelial relationships to the tooth surface where possible, and the minimization of areas of nonkeratinized marginal epithelium, especially in the presence of restorative dentistry.
4. The elimination of all other physical relationships that compromise patient and professional plaque-control measures. These include furcation involvements and subgingival restorative margins.
5. A clinically maintainable milieu. This condition will evolve as a result of the previous four criteria having been met.

Pocket-elimination therapy helps maintain the plaque-host equilibrium in the host's favor, by closing the window of host vulnerability due to characteristics of the periodontium as much as possible.

RATIONALE FOR POCKETING-ELIMINATION PROCEDURES USING OSSEOUS RESECTIVE TECHNIQUES

Periodontal pockets are recognized as complicating factors in thorough patient and professional plaque control. Waerhaug has shown that flossing and brushing are only effective to a depth of about 2.5 mm subgingivally (3). Beyond this depth, significant amounts of plaque remain attached to the root surface following a patient's oral hygiene procedures. Professional prophylaxis results are also compromised in the presence of deeper pockets. The failure of root planing to completely remove subgingival plaque and calculus in deeper pockets is well documented in the literature (4–8). Through the examination of extracted teeth, which had been root planed until they were judged plaque free by all available clinical parameters, Waerhaug (3) demonstrated that instrumentation of pockets measuring 3 mm or less was successful, with regard to total plaque removal, in 83% of the cases. In pockets of 3–5 mm in depth, 61% of the teeth exhibited retained plaque after thorough root planing. When pocket depths were 5 mm or more, failure to completely remove adherent plaque was the finding 89% of the time. Tabita et al. (9) noted that no tooth demonstrated a plaque-free surface 14 days after thorough root planing when the pretreatment pocket depths were 4–6 mm, even in the presence of excellent supragingival plaque control.

Such reinfection of a treated site occurs along three pathways (3, 9):

1. Plaque that remains in root lacunae, grooves, etc., multiplies and repopulates the root surface following therapy.
2. Plaque that is adherent to the epithelial lining of the pocket repopulates the root surface after healing. Complete removal of the epithelial lining of the pocket is not a common finding following curettage (10–12).
3. Supragingival plaque extends subgingivally, beyond the reach of the patient, and adheres to the root surface.

Waerhaug has stated, "If the pocket depth is more than 5 mm, the chances of failure are so great that there is an obvious indication for surgical pocket elimination" (3).

Poor soft-tissue morphologies contribute to increased plaque accumulation. Deep, sharp clefts and marked soft-tissue marginal discrepancies in adjacent areas are contributing factors to inadequate patient plaque control (13).

The morphology of the interproximal soft-tissue col must also be considered. When the buccal and/or lingual peaks of tissue are coronal to the contact point, the gingiva must "dip" under the contact point to reach the other side, resulting in a concave col form (14–16). Because the col tissue touches the contact point, its epithelium does not keratinize (17,18) (Fig. 1.54). Lack of keratinization is not an inherent property of either col or sulcular epithelium, as this tissue will keratinize when it is no longer in contact with the tooth, either as a result of periodontal therapy or eversion (18–20). Nonkeratinized epithelium is less resistant to disruption and penetration by bacterial plaque than its keratinized counterpart (21, 22). When a concave, nonkeratinized col form is present, the patient must try to control an area that is conducive to plaque accumulation and more

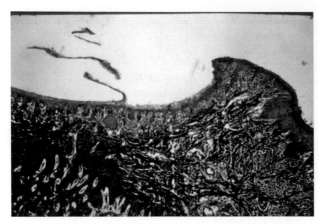

Fig. 1.54 The epithelium covering the soft tissues of the concave interproximal col form is not keratinized, due to the epithelium touching the contact points of the adjacent teeth. This nonkeratinized tissue is more vulnerable to penetration by bacterial by-products.

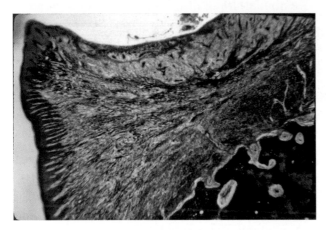

Fig. 1.55 The concave nonkeratinized col form demonstrates significant inflammation and tissue breakdown, as a result of its penetration by bacterial by-products.

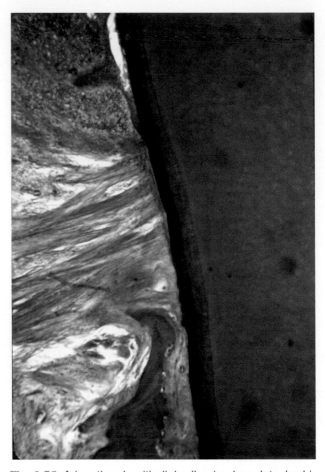

Fig. 1.56 A junctional epithelial adhesion has detached in the face of an inflammatory insult. Note that the connective tissue attachment is still intact apical to the inflammatory infiltrate.

easily breached by the plaque and its by-products (Fig. 1.55).

Junctional Epithelial Adhesion or Connective Tissue Attachment?

The tenuous nature of the epithelial adherence to the tooth and the ease with which it is separated from the root surface in the presence of inflammation are well known (23–29). The junctional epithelium represents a dual compromise, as it more easily penetrated by bacterial enzymes and more easily detached in the presence of inflammation than connective tissue fibers inserted into root cementum (Fig. 1.56). The "initial" periodontal lesion develops as follows:

1. Bacterial accumulation occurs in the gingival sulcus.
2. An increase in the concentration of specific bacterial products takes place.
3. These products penetrate the more permeable junctional epithelium, into the underlying connective tissue.
4. Dilation of the intercellular spaces of the junctional epithelium occurs and polymorphonuclear and mononuclear cells become present.
5. Perivascular collagen destruction takes place.
6. Progression to the "early" periodontal lesion occurs.

In light of its relative biologic and mechanical inferiority when compared to connective tissue attachment to the root surface, the expanse of junctional epithelial adhesion to the tooth should be minimized. This goal is accomplished through appropriate osseous resective surgery with apically positioned flaps. An attachment apparatus is formed, which consists of approximately one millimeter of connective tissue fiber insertion into the root surface, followed by one millimeter of junctional epithelial adhesion coronally (30,31). The connective tissue attachment is derived from a combination of outgrowth of the periodontal ligament and resorption of the osseous crest (32). This result is markedly different than the postsurgical attachment apparatus obtained following either curettage or replaced flap (modified Widman or open-flap curettage) surgery, which demonstrate healing to previously periodontally affected root surfaces by the formation of a long junctional epithelial adhesion (33–51). The length of the junctional epithelium is dependent upon the distance between the osseous crest and the margin of the soft tissue. In contrast, pocket-elimination surgery consistently results in a short junctional epithelium, avoiding the compromises inherent in a longer epithelial adhesive relationship.

The Significance of Furcation Involvements

Horizontal destruction of periodontal support, which results in furcation involvements, is a significant negative factor with regard to long-term prognosis if left untreated. The inaccessibility of even early furcation involvements to proper plaque control measures is well documented (4, 52–55). In addition, "maintenance" care, open and closed debridement, chemical treatment of the root surface, and placement of particulate materials without covering membranes have all failed to demonstrate predictable success in the treatment of the periodontally involved furcation. Removal of the vertical periodontal pocket without eliminating the horizontal component of a furcation involvement results in a compromised environment for the removal of plaque, and contributes to continued periodontal breakdown.

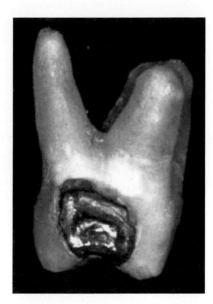

Fig. 1.57 Recurrent caries has developed at the most apical extent of a deep subgingival interproximal restoration.

The Influence of Restorative Margins

Restorative-margin position also influences long-term periodontal health, as plaque accumulation at the restorative-margin–tooth interface is a consistent finding, in both research and clinical practice (56–63). When a restorative margin extends subgingival, the resultant increased plaque accumulation often leads to acceleration of periodontal breakdown and recurrent caries (63, 64) (Fig. 1.57). This fact is especially critical if the attachment apparatus in place includes a long junctional epithelium, as the increased permeability and detachability of a long junctional epithelial adhesion in the face of inflammation lend the long junctional epithelium a greater vulnerability to the increased inflammatory insult inherent in subgingival margin placement.

Does Pocket-Elimination Therapy Work?

Smith et al. (65) and Olsen et al. (66) evaluated the relative efficacies of appropriately executed osseous resection with apically positioned flaps, and apically positioned flaps with root planing alone. Data were pooled by pocket depth and subdivided into tooth surfaces within a given pocket depth, to help elucidate the strengths and differences of the postsurgical attachment apparati. Mesial and distal probing depths were recorded with the probe placed as far interproximally as possible, and angulated to follow the long axis of the tooth. Only lesions that were amenable to resective therapy, and could therefore properly evaluate its applicability, were so treated. Surgical photographs were published, which demonstrated the techniques employed.

Five years postoperatively, statistically significant interproximal pocket-depth differences were noted between the sites treated with and without osseous resective therapy. Pocket depths in the flap curettage areas were approaching preoperative values, while the pocket elimination attained in other sites with osseous therapy was maintained. On the buccal and lingual surfaces, pocket elimination was maintained with both treatment approaches, underscoring both the fragility of a junctional epithelial adhesion and the danger of collapsing data. Radicularly, where patient plaque removal was easier and the junctional epithelium was shorter, pocket elimination was maintained following both types of therapies. However, in interproximal areas where plaque removal was more difficult and there was a longer junctional epithelial relationship to the root surface following root planing, curettage, and apically positioned flap therapy due to the presence of osseous craters, repocketing occurred in sites treated with open-flap curettage. Flap curettage sites that initially probed 4 mm underwent repocketing at 5 years three times more often than sites treated via osseous resection. If initial probing depths were 5 mm, flap-curettage sites repocketed 3.6 times as often as those treated with osseous resection. With initial probings of 6–8 mm, repocketing was six times as likely to occur with open-flap curettage. Bleeding upon probing was encountered 2.3 times more often in sites treated with open-flap curettage than those treated with osseous resection, 5 years postoperatively. As expected, there was a 91 % correlation between the presence of subgingival plaque and bleeding upon probing.

Lindhe and Nyman (67) reported the 14-year results of pocket-elimination therapy in 61 patients with advanced periodontal disease preoperatively, who had remained on regular maintenance schedules. Only 0.49 teeth were lost per patient over 14 years. Disease progression was shown to be 20–30 times slower than in Swedes with untreated periodontal disease (68).

Nabers et al. (69) reported upon the results of 1,435 patients treated via pocket-elimination therapy. Patients lost an average of 0.29 teeth per patient over a mean postoperative time of 12.9 years.

Retrospective studies that assess treatment modalities other than pocket-elimination therapy carried out in patients with active periodontal disease demonstrated markedly different results than those reported upon following use of pocket-elimination therapy.

McFall (70) reported an average tooth loss of 2.6 teeth per patient 19 years post-therapy; a ninefold greater tooth loss than that reported by Nabers et al. (69). Similarly, Goldman et al. (71) documented a tooth mortality rate of 3.6 teeth per patient 22.2 years post-active periodontal therapy. Such mortality represented an incidence of tooth loss approximately 13 times greater than that reported by Nabers et al.

Kaldahl et al. (72, 73) compared treatment results in 82 periodontal patients treated in a split mouth design with either root planing, modified Widman surgery, or flap surgery with osseous resection. Breakdown of sites during maintenance care of up to 7 years was greater in areas treated with modified Widman surgery and scaling and root planing than in areas treated with osseous resective therapy. These differences became more dramatic as initial pocket depth increased, underscoring the superiority of osseous resective therapy as a clinical modality for eliminating pockets and rendering areas maintainable over time by patients. Shallower pocket depths, coupled with the biologically stronger attachment apparatus of a short connective tissue attachment and a short junctional epithelium attained after osseous resection, proved more resistant to periodontal breakdown during maintenance than the attachment apparatus of a short connective tissue attachment and a long junctional epithelial adhesion obtained following root planing or modified Widman surgery.

Differences in tooth retention can be traced to the ability of the patient and the clinician to successfully and predictably effect thorough plaque removal. Properly performed pocket-elimination therapy provides an environment of minimal probing depth, which is conducive to plaque removal. Patient plaque removal is only effective to a subgingival depth of 2.5 mm (3). The clinician must not be misled by the supragingival scenario. Lindhe et al. (74) have demonstrated that there is no relationship between supragingival plaque control and changes in probing depths or attachment levels, or between supragingival plaque control and bleeding upon probing. Waerhaug spoke of the existence of subclinical inflammation (3). In such a situation, the tissues appear healthy, but periodontal destruction is occurring subgingivally.

Badersten et al. (75, 76) and Waite (77) noted that bleeding upon probing was directly related to pocket depth, with deeper areas bleeding more often. Therefore, the same limitations that apply to subgingival root planing in the face of pocket depths must be considered in the maintenance phase of therapy.

The deeper the residual probing depths, the more difficult debridement and maintenance become for both the patient and the dental professional (78–85). Sites with probing depths of greater than or equal to 6 mm are at significantly higher risk for future deterioration and additional attachment loss as a result of disease activity, if left untreated.

The scenario for continued loss of attachment in the face of post-therapeutic pocketing is as follows:

1. The patient presents with pocket depths in excess of 3 mm.
2. Patient plaque control removes plaque up to 2.5 mm subgingivally.
3. The attachment apparatus which results from curettage, modified Widman surgery, or flap curettage, has a long junctional epithelial component.
4. This epithelial adhesion exhibits greater permeability to plaque than a connective tissue fiber insertion.
5. Junctional epithelium is easily detached from the root in the presence of inflammation.
6. Subgingival scaling is increasingly less effective in areas probing greater than 3 mm.
7. Plaque left behind subgingivally following root planing begins to grow and repopulate the root surface within 14 days.
8. As the plaque front proceeds farther subgingivally, its removal is less effective.
9. As the pocket deepens, the problems with plaque removal are exacerbated.

10. The presence of furcation involvements and/or subgingival restorations makes plaque removal even more difficult.
11. The result is continued periodontal breakdown.

Employed in conjunction with selective extractions, root resective therapy, and prosthetic reconstruction, pocket-elimination techniques afford a high degree of predictability (86).

CLINICAL EXAMPLE SIX

A 26-year-old female presented in 1981 with a number of periodontal and restorative concerns. Postorthodontic blunting of the roots was noted (Fig. 1.58). Class I furcation involvements were present on all maxillary and mandibular molars. Subgingival caries was present in many areas. Osseointegrating implants were not a viable treatment option at the time of patient examination.

The combination of the patient's young age, short residual root structures, and active periodontal and restorative pathologies mandated a comprehensive, coordinated effort in order to afford her a predictable treatment outcome. The performance of periodontal surgical therapies that would not eliminate deeper pockets and furcation involvements and render all caries and defective

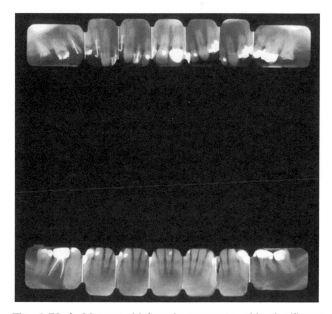

Fig. 1.58 A 26-year-old female presents with significant subgingival caries, Class I furcation involvements, and short roots on all maxillary teeth.

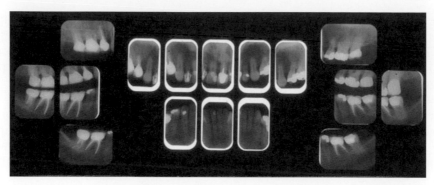

Fig. 1.59 Twenty-five years following appropriate periodontal and restorative therapy, all teeth have been maintained.

restorative margins supragingival for the restorative dentist's intervention would be ill-advised. When treating such a patient, the clinician has "one shot" at restoring the patient to health. The patient's limited attachment apparati could not withstand multiple surgical insults, nor afford to be subjected to continued periodontal breakdown following active care.

After ensuring the appropriate level of patient compliance with regard to plaque control efforts, the patient was treated with an osseous resective approach. All furcation involvements were eliminated through ondontoplasty. Tissues were positioned in such a manner as to allow placement of restorative margins supragingivally or intracrevicularly. The necessary restorative therapy was carried out.

A full series of radiographs taken 25 years after active therapy had been completed demonstrate the maintenance of periodontal support around the teeth, and the high degree of predictability afforded this patient through appropriate, coordinated care (Fig. 1.59).

Conclusion

When utilized appropriately, a multidisciplinary periodontal restorative approach is highly effective in the management of a variety of situations. Simple and complex patients may be successfully treated, with success being defined as long-term stability and maximization of patient comfort, function, and aesthetics. The challenge that will be discussed in subsequent chapters is how best to attain such treatment outcomes in everyday clinical practice.

References

1. Amsterdam M. Periodontal prosthesis: 25 years in retrospect. Alpha Omega 1974;67:8–52.
2. Fugazzotto PA. Implant and regenerative therapy in dentistry: A guide to decision making. Hoboken, NJ: Wiley-Blackwell Publishing, 2009.
3. Waerhaug J. Healing of the dento-epithelial junction following subgingival plaque control. II: As observed on extracted teeth. J Periodontol 1978;49:119–34.
4. Stambaugh RV, Dragoo M, Smith DM, Carosali L. The limits of subgingival scaling. Int J Periodontics Restorative Dent 1981;1:30–42.
5. Buchanan S, Robertson P. Calculus removal by scaling/root planing with and without surgical access. J Periodontol 1987;58:159.
6. Jones WA, O'Leary TJ. The effectiveness of root planing in removing bacterial endotoxin from the roots of periodontally involved teeth. J Periodontol 1978;49:337–42.
7. Rabbani GM, Ash MM, Caffesse RG. The effectiveness of subgingival scaling and root planing in calculus removal. J Periodontol 1981;52:119–23.
8. Caffesse R, Sweeney PL, Smith BA. Scaling and root planing with and without periodontal flap surgery. J Clin Periodontol 1986;13:205–10.
9. Tabita PV, Bissada NF, Maybury JE. Effectiveness of supragingival plaque control on the development of subgingival plaque and gingival inflammation in patients with moderate pocket depth. J Periodontol 1981;52:88–93.
10. Waerhaug J, Steen E. The presence or absence of bacteria in the gingival pocket and the reaction in healthy pockets to certain pure cultures. Odont Tidsk 1952;60:1–24.
11. Stahl SS. Healing of gingival tissues following various therapeutic regimens—A review of histologic studies. J Oral Ther and Pharm 1965;2:145–60.
12. Morris M. The removal of pocket and attachment epithelium in humans: A histologic study. J Periodontol 1954;25:7–11.

13. Smukler HM, Landsberg J. The toothbrush and gingival traumatic injury. J Periodontol 1984;55:713–19.
14. Nevins M. Interproximal periodontal disease—the embrasure as an etiologic factor. Int J Periodontics Restorative Dent 1982;2:9–27.
15. Fugazzotto PA. Preparation of the periodontium for restorative dentistry. St Louis: Ishiyaku EuroAmerica, 1989:44–54.
16. Ochsenbein C. A primer for osseous surgery. Int J Periodontics Restorative Dent 1986;6:8–46.
17. Johnson RL. Osseous surgery in periodontal therapy. In: Prichard JF, ed., The diagnosis and treatment of periodontal disease in general dental practice. Philadelphia: The W. B. Saunders Co., 1979.
18. Fugazzotto PA, Parma-Benfenati S. Preprosthetic periodontal considerations. Crown length and biologic width. Quint Internat 1984;15:1247–56.
19. Gelfand HB, Tencate AR, Freeman E. The keratinization potential of crevicular epithelium: An experimental study. J Periodontol 1978;49:113–18.
20. Caffesse RG, Karring T, Nasjleti CE. Keratinizing potential of sulcular epithelium. J Periodontol 1977;48:140–46.
21. Caffesse RG, Nasjleti CE. Enzymatic penetration through intact sulcular epithelium. J Periodontol 1976;47:391–97.
22. Thilander H. The effect of leukocytic enzymes activity on the structure of the gingival pocket epithelium in man. Acta Odont Scand 1963;21:431–51.
23. Listgarten MA. Similarity of epithelial relationships in the gingiva of rat and man. J Periodontol 1975;46:677–80.
24. Listgarten MA. Periodontal probing: What does it mean? J Clin Periodontol 1980;7:165–76.
25. Saglie R, Johansen JR, Flotra L. The zone of completely and partially destructed periodontal fibers in pathological pockets. J Clin Periodontol 1975;2:198–202.
26. Spray JR, Garnick JJ, Doles LR, Klawitter JJ. Microscopic demonstration of the position of periodontal probes. J Periodontol 1978;49:148–52.
27. Silvertson JF, Burgett FG. Probing of pockets related to the attachment level. J Periodontol 1976;47:281–86.
28. Powell B, Garnick JJ. The use of extracted teeth to evaluate clinical measurements of periodontal disease. J Periodontol 1978;49:621–24.
29. Spray R, Garnick JJ. Position of probes in human periodontal pockets. J Dent Res 1979;58(Special Issue A),176. Abstract No. 331.
30. Ruben MP, Schulman SM, Kon S. Healing of periodontal surgical wounds. In: Goldman HM, Cohen DW, eds. Periodontal therapy. 5th ed. St Louis: CV Mosby Company, 1973.
31. Parma-Benfenati S, Fugazzotto PA, Ruben MP. The effect of restorative margins on the postsurgical development and nature of the periodontium. Int J Periodontics Restorative Dent 1985;5:31–51.
32. Carnevale G, Sterrantino SF, DiFebo G. Soft and hard tissue wound healing following tooth preparation to the alveolar crest. Int J Periodontics Restorative Dent 1983;3:37–53.
33. Vieira E, O'Leary T, Kafrawy A. The effect of sodium hypochlorite and citric acid solutions on healing of periodontal pockets. J Periodontol 1982;53:71–80.
34. Caton J, Nyman S, Zander H. Histometric evaluation of periodontal surgery II. Connective tissue attachment levels after four regenerative procedures. J Clin Periodontol 1980;7:224–31.
35. Kalkwarf K, Tussing G, Davis M. Histologic evaluation of gingival curettage facilitated by sodium hypochlorite solution. J Periodontol 1982;53:63–70.
36. Yukna R. A clinical and histologic study of healing following the Excisional New Attachment Procedure in Rhesus monkeys. J Periodontol 1976;47:701–9.
37. Yukna R, Lawrence J. Gingival surgery for soft tissue new attachment. Dent Clin N Amer 1980;24:705–18.
38. Bowen W, Bowers G, Bergquist J, Organ R. Removal of pocket epithelium in humans utilizing an internally beveled incision. Int J Periodontics Restorative Dent 1981;1:9–19.
39. Froum W, Coran J, Thaller B, et al. Periodontal healing following open debridement flap procedures. I. Clinical assessment of soft tissue and osseous repair. J Periodontol 1982;53:8–14.
40. Caton J, Zander H. Osseous repair of an infrabony pocket without new attachment of connective tissue. J Clin Periodontol 1976;47:54–62.
41. Hiatt W, Schallhorn R, Aaronian A. The induction of new bone and cementum formation. IV. Microscopic examination of the periodontium following human bone and marrow allograft, autograft, and nongraft periodontal regeneration procedures. J Periodontol 1978;49:495–512.
42. Egelberg J. Regeneration and repair of periodontal tissues. J Periodont Res 1987;22:233–42.
43. Wirthlin MR. The current status of new attachment therapy. J Periodontol 1981;52:529–44.
44. Listgarten M, Rosenberg M. Histological study of repair following new attachment procedures in human periodontal lesions. J Periodontol 1979;50:333–44.
45. Ellagaard B, Karring T, Listgarten M, Loe H. New attachment after treatment of interradicular lesions. J Periodontol 1973;44:209–17.
46. Stahl S, Froum S, Kushner L. Periodontal healing following open debridement flap procedures. II. Histologic observations. J Periodontol 1982;53:15–21.
47. Frank R, Fiore-Donno G, Cimasoni G, Matter J. Ultrastructural study of epithelial and connective tissue

gingival reattachment in man. J Periodontol 1974;45: 626–35.

48. Stahl S. Repair or regeneration. J Clin Periodontol 1979; 6:389–96.

49. Magnusson I, Ronstad L, Nyman S, Lindhe J. A long junctional epithelium—A locus minoris resistentiae in plaque infection? J Clin Periodontol 1983;10:333–40.

50. Beaumont R, O'Leary T, Kafrawy A. Relative resistance of long junctional epithelial adhesions and connective tissue attachments to plaque-induced inflammation. J Periodontol 1984;55:213–25.

51. Caton J, Nyman S. Histometric evaluation of periodontal surgery. I. The modified Widman flap procedure. J Clin Periodontol 1980;7:212–23.

52. Ross I, Thompson R. Furcation involvement in maxillary and mandibular molars. J Periodontol 1980;51:450–54.

53. Larato DC. Some anatomical factors related to furcation involvements. J Periodontol 1975;46:608–9.

54. Ricchetti PA. A furcation classification based on pulp chamber–furcation relationships and vertical radiographic bone loss. Int J Periodontics Restorative Dent 1982;2:51–59.

55. Sternlicht HC. New approach to the management of multirooted teeth with advanced periodontal disease. J Periodontol 1963;34:150–58.

56. Karlsen K. Gingival reaction to dental restorations. Acta Odont Scand 1970;28:895–99.

57. Waerhaug J. Tissue reactions around artificial crowns. J Periodontol 1953;24:172–85.

58. Newcomb GM. The relationship between the location of subgingival crown margins and gingival inflammation. J Periodontol 1974;45:151–54.

59. Renggli HH, Regolati B. Gingival inflammation and plaque accumulation by well adapted supragingival and subgingival proximal restorations. Helv Odontol Acta 1972;16:99–101.

60. Waerhaug J. Effect of rough surfaces upon gingival tissues. J Dent Res 1956;35:323–25.

61. Silness J. Periodontal conditions in patients treated with dental bridges. II. The influence of full and partial crowns on plaque accumulation, development of gingivitis and pocket formation. J Perio Res 1970;5:219–24.

62. Mormann W, Regolatti B, Renggli HH. Gingival reaction to well fitted subgingival gold inlays. J Clin Periodontol 1974;1:120–25.

63. Gilmore N, Sheiham A. Overhanging dental restorations and periodontal disease. J Periodontol 1971;42:8–12.

64. Fugazzotto PA. Periodontal restorative interrelationships: The isolated restoration. J Amer Dent Assoc 1985;110:915–17.

65. Smith DH, Ammons WF, van Belle G. A longitudinal study of periodontal status comparing flap curettage and osseous recontouring. I. Six month results. J Periodontol 1980;51:367–75.

66. Olsen CT, Ammons WF, van Belle G. A longitudinal study comparing apically repositioned flaps, with and without osseous surgery. Int J Periodontics Restorative Dent 1985;5:11–33.

67. Lindhe J, Nyman S. Long term maintenance of patients treated for advanced periodontal disease. J Clin Periodontol 1984;11:504–14.

68. Lindhe J, Haffajee AD, Socransky SS. Progression of periodontal disease in adult subjects in the absence of periodontal therapy. J Clin Periodontol 1983;10:433–42.

69. Nabers CL, Stalker WH, Esparza D, Naylor B, Canales S. Tooth loss in 1535 treated periodontal patients. J Periodontol 1988;59:297–300.

70. McFall WT. Tooth loss in 100 treated patients with periodontal disease. A long term study. J Periodontol 1982;53:539–49.

71. Goldman M, Ross I, Goteiner D. Effect of periodontal therapy on patients maintained for 15 years or longer: A retrospective study. J Periodontol 1986;57:347–53.

72. Kaldahl W B, Kalkwarf K L, Kashinath D P, Molvar M P, Dyer J K. Long term evaluation of periodontal therapy: I. Response to four therapeutic modalities. J Periodontol 1996;67:93–102.

73. Kaldahl W B, Kalkwarf K L, Kashinath D P, Molvar M P, Dyer J K. Long term evaluation of periodontal therapy: II. Incidence of sites breaking down. J Periodontol 1996;67:103–8.

74. Lindhe J, Okamoto H, Yoneyama T, Haffajee A, Socransky SS. Longitudinal changes in periodontal disease in untreated subjects. J Clin Periodontol 1989;16:662–70.

75. Badersten A, Nilveus R, Egelberg J. Effect of nonsurgical periodontal therapy. II. Severely advanced periodontitis. J Clin Periodontol 1984;11:63–76.

76. Badersten A, Nilveus R, Egelberg J. Effect of nonsurgical periodontal therapy. III. Single versus repeated instrumentation. J Clin Periodontol 1984;11:114–24.

77. Waite IM. A comparison between conventional gingivectomy and a nonsurgical regime in the treatment of periodontitis. J Clin Periodontol 1976;3:173–85.

78. Buchanan SA, Robertson PB. Calculus removal by scaling/root planing with and without surgical access. J Periodontol 1987;58:159–63

79. Rabbani GM, Ash MM, Caffesse RG. The effectiveness of subgingival scaling and root planing in calculus removal. J Periodontol 1981;52:119–23.

80. Waerhaug J. Healing of the dental epithelial junction following subgingival plaque control. II: As observed on extracted teeth. J Periodontol 1978;49:119–34.

81. Jeffcoat MK, Reddy MS. Progression of probing attachment loss in adult periodontitis. J Peridontol 1991;62:185–89.

82. Badersten A, Nilveus R, Egelberg J. Effect of non-surgical periodontal therapy. VII. Bleeding, suppuration and probing depth in sites with probing attachment loss. J Clin Periodontol 1985:12:432–40.

83. Grbic J T, Lamstr I B. Risk indicators for future clinical attachment loss in adult periodontitis. Tooth and site variables. J Periodontol 1992;63:262–69.

84. Haffajee A D, Socransay S S, Smith C, Divart S. Microbial risk indicators for periodontal attachment loss. J Periodont Res 1991;26:293–96.

85. Vanooteghem R, Hutchenes L H, Garrett S, Kiger R, Egelberg J. Bleeding on probing and probing depth as indicators of the response to plaque control and root debridement. J Clin Periodontol 1987;14:226–30.

86. Rosenberg MM, Kay HB, Keough BE, Holt RL. Periodontal and prosthetic management for advanced cases. Chicago: Quintessence 1988:148–56.

Chapter 2
The Role of Crown-Lengthening Therapy

Paul Fugazzotto

In an effort to deliver high-quality, predictable restorative dentistry to patients, all treating practitioners must consider the dynamic interplay of tooth restoration, the restorative procedure itself, and the health of the surrounding hard and soft tissues. Every restoration, whether it be a Class II amalgam or a full-mouth fixed reconstruction, places added demands on the supporting periodontium (Figs. 2.1, 2.2). The most ideal marginal adaptation results in increased plaque accumulation at the restorative margin-tooth interface. Poorly contoured restorations will inhibit proper plaque control procedures, thus hastening periodontal breakdown and recurrent caries at the restorative margin-tooth interface (Figs. 2.3–2.6). Should such margins be placed subgingivally, the destructive process is accelerated by the inability of the patient to adequately carry out plaque control measures.

While many practitioners speak of the "self-cleansing zone" below the gingival margin, and the maintainability of a subgingival restoration if monitored carefully (1), Waerhaug has shown that even a well-fitting restoration will harbor plaque and bacteria (2).

Several clinical investigators have demonstrated the detrimental effects of poorly finished and/or incorrectly positioned restorations with subgingival margins on the periodontal tissues. Local gingival inflammation and loss of periodontal attachment are the results of such therapy (3–7). It has additionally been demonstrated that it is plaque accumulation in relation to an overhanging restorative margin, and not merely the subgingival restoration, that causes promotion of the periodontal disease process (7–9).

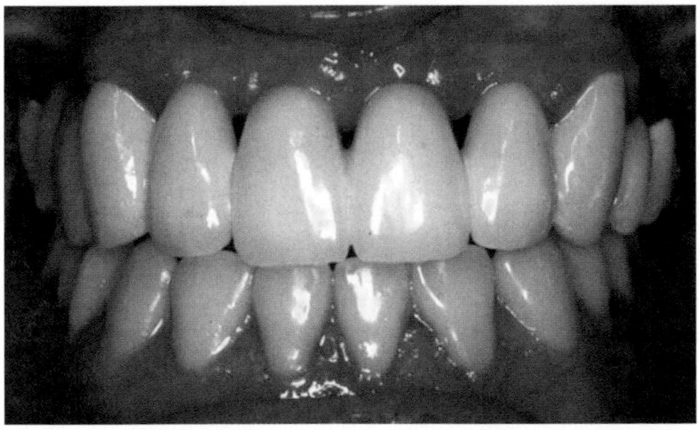

Fig. 2.1 Twenty-three years after restoration, a patient presents with a 14-unit maxillary fixed prosthesis supported by two first molars and two cuspids, and a mandibular overdenture retained by two cuspid roots with attachments. Such a successful therapeutic outcome requires an understanding and management of periodontal restorative interrelationships.

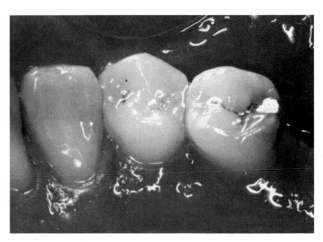

Fig. 2.2 Periodontal restorative interrelationships must also be appropriately understood and managed when placing an isolated Class II restoration on a tooth.

Periodontal Restorative Interrelationships: Ensuring Clinical Success, First Edition. Edited by Paul A. Fugazzotto.
© 2011 by John Wiley & Sons, Inc. Published 2011 by John Wiley & Sons, Inc.

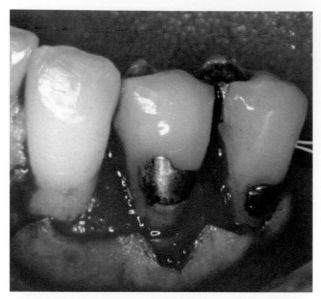

Fig. 2.3 Flap reflection reveals significant plaque and calculus accumulation at the restorative margin tooth interface, where the restoration extended subgingivally.

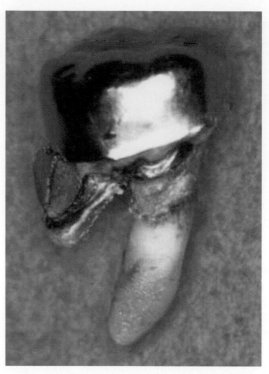

Fig. 2.4 A poor understanding of the periodontal ramifications of ill fitting restorative dentistry has led to the demise of a first molar. An aluminum shell crown was placed; subsequent decay developed at the restorative margin tooth interface and was repaired with a subgingival amalgam; the situation was not conducive to home-care efforts and continued plaque and calculus accumulation resulted in periodontal bone loss and additional caries on the distal root of the tooth; another restoration was placed, extending deeper subgingival. The net result was loss of the tooth.

Nowhere is the delicate balance of the restored tooth and the health of the surrounding periodontium more evident than in the restoration of an interproximal area. A multitude of factors—periodontal, restorative, and geometric in nature—work together to render this a primary area of concern in the successful management of any dentition compromised by oral bacteria. To properly manage the embrasure space, the area must be visualized as the fluid, three-dimensional entity it is.

Management of the Apico-occlusal Dimension

The concept of biologic width is paramount in understanding the apico-occlusal relationship of the restorative margin to the osseous crest. Proceeding coronally from the osseous crest, the attachment apparatus consists of Sharpey fiber insertion into the root surface, followed by a junctional epithelial adhesion to root surface, followed by the gingival sulcus (Fig. 2.7). The combined dimensions of the connective tissue and junctional epithelium are, on average, 2.04 mm in humans (10). Impingement upon this dimension by the restorative margin results in soft-tissue inflammation and eventual periodontal break down. In

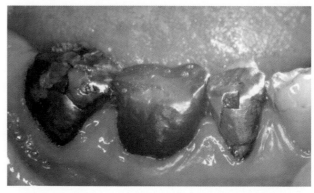

Fig. 2.5 A patient presents with older restorations which extend subgingivally. The tissues appear firm and pink. No clinical evidence of inflammation exists.

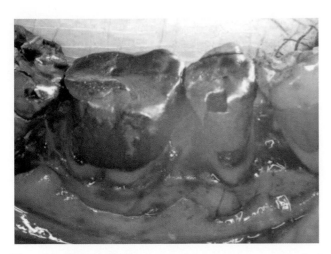

Fig. 2.6 Flap reflection reveals extensive subgingival caries around all restorations. Note the developing furcation involvement on the first molar, due in large part to the nonideal morphology of the subgingival restoration in the area. Failure to intervene in an appropriate, timely manner has resulted in poor prognoses for these teeth.

addition, postsurgical healing of tissues is impaired in the face of a compromised biologic width.

VIOLATING THE BIOLOGIC WIDTH

Violation of the biologic width can occur due to tooth preparation, which may damage the junctional epithelium and the supra-alveolar connective tissues. A progressive inflammatory process may also occur following soft tissue retraction procedures, various impression techniques, electrosurgery (Fig. 2.8), and the placement of a temporary restoration.

Fortunately, Löe and Silness have shown that injuries created by insertion of a retraction cord are reversible, as long as the lesions are allowed to heal against a clean tooth surface (11). Duncan (12) found that damage attributed to poorly contoured provisional restorations was reversible, as long as the provisional restorations were modified and placed correctly. However, if inflammation occurs and is not resolved, the inflammatory process is perpetuated when the final restoration is cemented in the previously injured and inflamed area (13). Irreversible damage results, characterized by the development of a periodontal pocket, with apical migration of the junctional epithelium and loss of attachment. Placement of restorations prior to total healing and development of the supracrestal

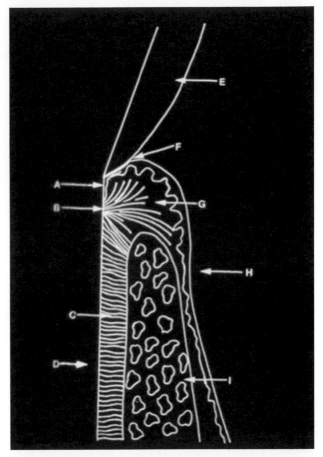

Fig. 2.7 A diagrammatic representation of a healthy attachment apparatus. A = junctional epithelium; B = supracrestal connective tissue insertion; C = periodontal ligament; D = root; E = enamel; F = gingival sulcus; G = gingival connective tissue; H = covering epithelium; I = alveolar bone.

attachment apparatus postsurgically is also highly problematic, as it is impossible to know in advance where the most coronal position of the attachment apparatus will be (Fig. 2.9). The net result is violation of the biologic width, impingement upon the attachment apparatus and development of an inflammatory lesion.

Studies by Fugazzotto and Parma-Benfenati (14) and Parma-Benfenati et al. (15) examined the effects of restorative margin positions on the development and health of the supracrestal attachment apparatus postsurgically, as well as the role that quantity and quality of alveolar housing played in such attachment apparatus development. At the control sites, Class V amalgam restorations were placed 4 mm coronal to the osseous crest in beagle dogs, and the teeth were notched at the

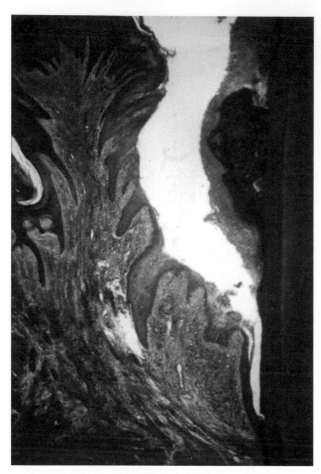

Fig. 2.8 Injudicious use of electrosurgery has resulted in irreversible damage to the root surface and the attachment apparatus. Note the inflammatory lesion in the soft tissues, the damaged root cementum, and the loss of periodontal attachment to the tooth.

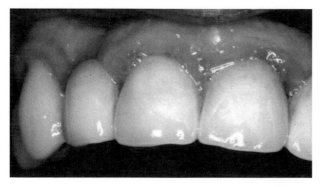

Fig. 2.9 Following periodontal osseous surgery, impressions were taken and full coverage restorations were fabricated and inserted prior to development and maturation of the supracrestal attachment apparatus. Note the inflamed, rolled nature of the marginal soft tissues.

osseous crest. In the experimental sites, Class V amalgam restorations were placed at osseous crest.

Histological examination 12 weeks posttherapy underscored the effects of restorative margin position on postsurgical attachment apparatus development. At the control sites, all tissues healed uneventfully. Histologic specimens were characterized by connective tissue reattachment to the root surface supracrestally for approximately 1 mm, followed by 1–1.5 mm of junctional epithelial adhesion. Minimal alveolar bone crest resorption was evident (Figs. 2.10, 2.11). This crestal resorption was more pronounced in specimens where thinner preoperative bone had been present.

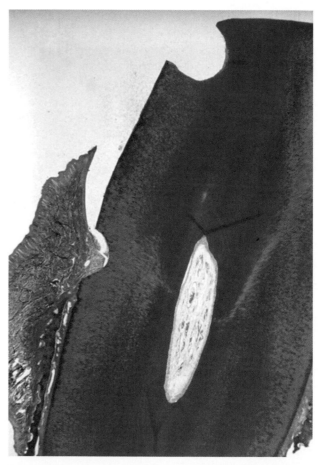

Fig. 2.10 In control sites, an amalgam restoration was placed at least 4 mm coronal to the crestal bone, and the root surface was notched at the crestal bone at the time of periodontal flap surgery. A 12-week postoperative histologic specimen demonstrates no signs of inflammation, and a healthy periodontal attachment apparatus crestal to the alveolar bone.

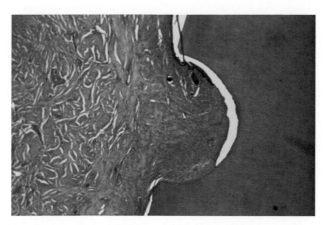

Fig. 2.11 A close-up of the notched area of the root demonstrates connective tissue attachment and a lack of inflammatory cells in control sites.

In the experimental sites, the tissues coronal to the restoration were characterized by a thin atrophic epithelial lining, which was not attached to the root surface, and a localized inflammatory reaction in the gingival soft tissues. This epithelium extended slightly apical to the restoration (Figs. 2.12–2.14). In all histological specimens of experimental sites, bone resorption was present to a varying degree, depending upon the quantity and quality of the preoperative bony septum. Thinner preoperative septa demonstrated greater loss of bone height than their thicker counterparts. Connective tissue attachment to the root surface always occurred apical to the restoration following the bone loss.

Clinically, the healed tissues in the control sites appeared healthy and did not bleed upon probing. The postoperative tissues at the experimental sites demonstrated significant clinical inflammation and bleeding upon probing.

The study demonstrated that:

1. Following surgical intervention, osseous resorption occurs. This pattern of resorption is influenced by the preoperative bone morphology.
2. When the biologic width is violated, inflammation not only will result in osseous resorption in an attempt to afford space for connective tissue insertion into the root supracrestally, but also will perpetuate the ongoing pathological process.
3. The presence of subgingival restorations will result in greater plaque accumulation.

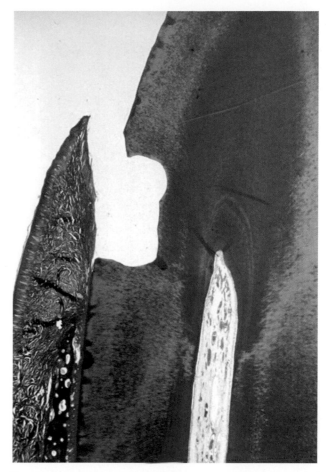

Fig. 2.12 In experimental sites, a restoration was placed at the alveolar crest during periodontal flap surgery. A 12-week histologic specimen demonstrates significant loss of alveolar crest height, apical positioning of the connective tissue insertion into the root, and ulcerated, inflamed tissues over the restoration.

4. Histologically, the findings adjacent to a subgingival restoration will correspond to those encountered when examining an inflammatory periodontal lesion.
5. When a restoration impinges upon the needed dimensions for development of the attachment apparatus during healing after periodontal surgical therapy, the extent of osseous loss encountered will be greater than when such a compromise is not present.
6. When a subgingival restoration is present, the inflammatory lesion encountered in the healed periodontal tissues postsurgically will be walled off by the establishment of a new "dentoperiosteal" fiber system. This

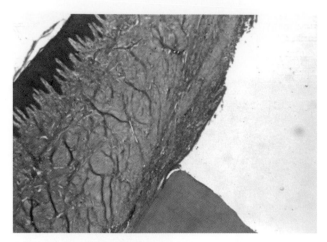

Fig. 2.13 The epithelium is thin or nonexistent in the experimental site. A heavy inflammatory infiltrate is noted in the gingival connective tissue.

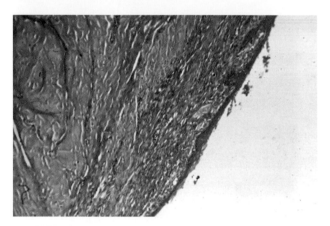

Fig. 2.14 A close-up demonstrates the ulcerated epithelium in the area of the restoration. Note the significant inflammatory infiltrate in the gingival connective tissue.

"dentoperiosteal" fiber system will be more apical than it would be if the restoration were not present, and will occur in the presence of greater loss of osseous structures crestally.

In light of the fact that a continuing inflammatory lesion is present when a subgingival restoration exists that impinges upon the necessary dimensions for reestablishment of a healthy attachment apparatus postsurgically, and because this attachment apparatus will establish itself regardless of osseous loss, crown-lengthening procedures to establish adequate biologic width to ensure that restorations are not placed too close to the osseous crest are usually justifiable.

In situations where the septa consisted of both thin and thick components, the thinner portions of the septa were resorbed to a greater extent. These findings are in agreement with widely accepted understanding regarding postsurgical periodontal healing. Ruben et al. (16) postulated that thinner septa would demonstrate greater liability than their thicker counterparts due to their biological and histological characteristics. Thin bony septa predominantly consist of cortical plates with a small marrow component. As a result, such septa are deficient in their primary source of pluripotential cells, which have the ability to differentiate into blastic cells of both hard- and soft-tissue natures. Thus, the osteogenic reaction expected following initial postsurgical resorption is attenuated or absent altogether in the presence of thin osseous septa. The initial resorptive phase itself may often be enough to eliminate a thin osseous septum because of its buccolingual dimension.

Parma-Benfenati et al. (14,16) found this to be the case in most of the thin septal specimens examined. The osseous septum began to resorb progressively from the external aspect of the septum inward (i.e., from the periosteal aspect toward the periodontal ligament). Simultaneously, resorption occurred from its thin coronal aspects. As the septum resorbed in the presence of the postsurgical chronic inflammatory process which is associated with any surgical procedure, the bone was replaced by connective tissues. These connective tissues served to join the periosteum with the remaining components of the periodontal ligament, which remained inserted into the cementum of the tooth (17).

When thicker bony septa had been present preoperatively, the biological and histological characteristics of the postoperative bone, and hence the postoperative results, were markedly different. Thicker septa contain greater amounts of marrow components than their thinner counterparts, and are thus capable of a more exuberant osteogenic response to surgical insult. When the cortical plate is resorbed, a pluripotential cell population is unmasked, yielding the expected result of new bone and other tissues. A highly exaggerated initial resorptive phase would be necessary to result in the obliteration of a thick bony septum. As a result, significantly less occluso-apical osseous loss was found when thick bony septa were present preoperatively, as compared to thin bony septa specimens.

Prior to the work of Parma-Benfenati et al. (14,15), no well-controlled clinical or histological studies had been performed that compared the extent and pattern of osseous resorption following a given surgical procedure in a thin septal scenario to that of a thicker septal scenario. Authors had discussed these considerations following gingival autograft placement (18,19). Friedman has shown that 0.5 mm of osseous resorption occurred during healing following osseous resective surgery when a thick bone septum was present, but did not compare his findings to those when a thin bony septum was present presurgically (20).

CROWN-LENGTHENING SURGERY

Although specific instances exist where nothing more than recontouring of the soft tissues is necessary to affect appropriate crown-lengthening osseous surgery, such a clinical scenario is infrequent. Rather, osseous resective therapy is usually required, in conjunction with appropriate soft-tissue management, to expose the desired clinical crown, ensure the development of an appropriate post-therapeutic attachment apparatus, and help establish the most ideal milieu for reception of the planned restorative dentistry.

CLINICAL EXAMPLE ONE

A patient presents with subgingival recurrent caries around an amalgam "patch" which had previously been placed to treat recurrent caries around a gold crown. The amalgam restoration extends deep subgingival (Fig. 2.15).

Flap reflection demonstrates the nonideal contours of the amalgam patch that had previously been placed (Fig. 2.16). Note the recurrent caries on the distal aspect of the subgingival extension of the amalgam patch, and the plaque trap that has been created in the furcation area. Failure to intervene appropriately would result in a poor prognosis for the first molar. Following recontouring of the amalgam restoration to eliminate its nonideal contours and appropriate osseous resective therapy, the buccal mucoperiosteal flap is sutured at osseous crest with interrupted gut 4-0 silk sutures (Fig. 2.17). Eight weeks postoperatively, the tissues have healed well, there is no evidence of a buccal furcation involvement, and the recurrent caries is exposed and accessible for appropriate restoration

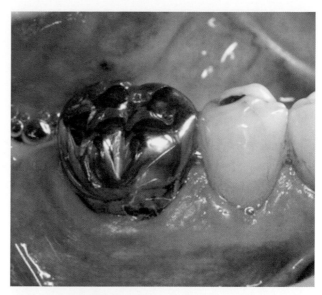

Fig. 2.15 A patient presents with recurrent subgingival caries around an amalgam "patch" on a first molar.

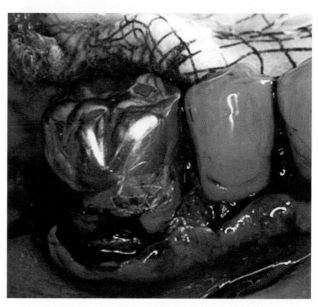

Fig. 2.16 Following flap reflection, recurrent caries around the amalgam restoration is evident. Note the "furcation involvement" due to the inability to appropriately contour the amalgam restoration deep subgingivally.

and subsequent patient plaque control measures (Fig. 2.18).

CLINICAL EXAMPLE TWO

A patient presents with numerous older subgingival restorations and recurrent subgingival caries on

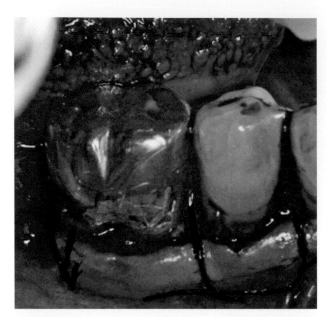

Fig. 2.17 Following appropriate osseous crown-lengthening surgery and reshaping of the amalgam restoration, the flaps are sutured at osseous crest with interrupted silk sutures.

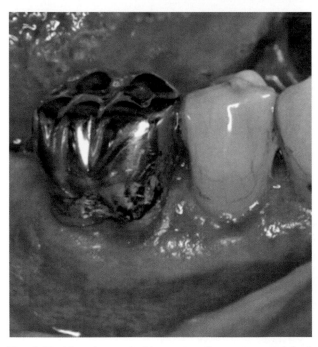

Fig. 2.18 All caries and older restorations are supragingival and accessible for appropriate restorative intervention following healing.

the mesiopalatal aspect of the maxillary first molar, and the palatal aspect of the maxillary first premolar (Fig. 2.19). Following appropriate flap design and reflection, including thinning and crestal anticipation of the palatal mucoperiosteal flap followed by the necessary osseous resective therapy, the buccal and palatal mucoperiosteal flaps are sutured at osseous crest with interrupted 4-0 silk sutures (Fig. 2.20). Eight weeks postoperatively, all subgingival restorations and/or recurrent caries are exposed and accessible for both appropriate restorative intervention and subsequent patient plaque-control efforts (Fig. 2.21).

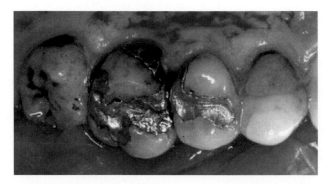

Fig. 2.19 A patient presents with older restorations, recurrent subgingival caries on the mesial palatal aspect of the maxillary first molar, and recurrent caries on the palatal aspect of the first premolar.

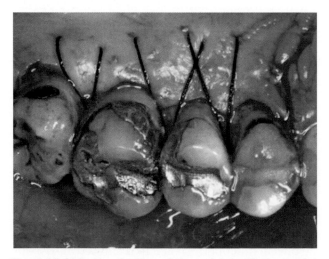

Fig. 2.20 Note the position of the palatal soft tissues following appropriate flap design and reflection, including crestal anticipation, osseous resection, and suturing with interrupted 4-0 silk sutures.

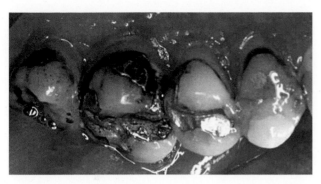

Fig. 2.21 Following appropriate crown-lengthening osseous surgery, all recurrent caries and older restorations are accessible for restorative intervention.

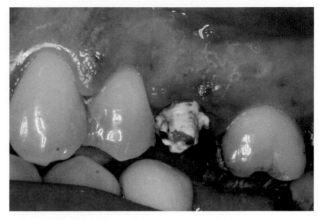

Fig. 2.23 Following removal of the provisional restoration, it is obvious that inadequate clinical tooth structure is present for appropriate reception of restorative therapy. Note the inflamed and nonideally shaped interproximal soft tissues.

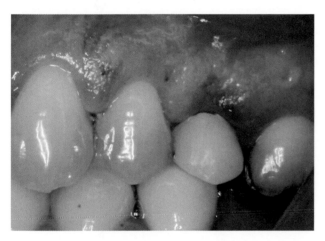

Fig. 2.22 A patient presents with a provisional restoration on the maxillary second premolar. Note the inflamed nature of the surrounding soft tissues.

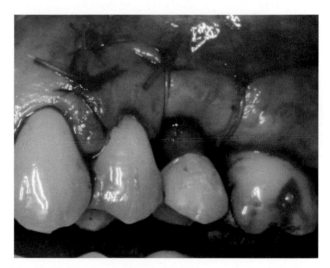

Fig. 2.24 Crown-lengthening osseous surgery has been performed, and the buccal and palatal flaps have been sutured at the alveolar osseous crest with interrupted plain gut sutures.

CLINICAL EXAMPLE THREE

A patient presents with a temporary full coverage restoration on the maxillary second premolar. Following removal of the temporary restoration, inadequate clinical crown length is present for appropriate restorative intervention. Crown-lengthening osseous surgery is performed in the manner already described, exposing adequate tooth structure and establishing biologic width. Following healing, the soft-tissue margin of the crown-lengthened tooth and the adjacent teeth are confluent and easily cleansable. More than adequate tooth structure is now exposed for appropriate restorative intervention (Figs. 2.22–2.24).

CLINICAL EXAMPLE FOUR

A patient presents with marked incomplete passive eruption and a problem with retention of the final full coverage restorations on her maxillary first and second premolars. Incomplete passive eruption will be subsequently discussed. The restorative dentist has attempted to improve retention of the restorations utilizing various permutations of grooves and pins in the prepared teeth. Periodontal crown-lengthening osseous surgery is carried out in the previously described manner, eliminating the incomplete passive eruption that is present and exposing adequate tooth structure for fabrication of restorations with ideal contours and the necessary retention. Following healing, more than adequate tooth structure is exposed for such therapeutic intervention. The final restorations demonstrate the desired restorative contours. No problem has been encountered with the retention of the final restorations (Figs. 2.25–2.28).

All too often, a discussion of crown-lengthening osseous surgery focuses immediately and almost exclusively upon osseous resection to establish the desired dimension between the alveolar crest and the planned restorative margin. Such focus, with the exclusion of other considerations, is ill-advised. Any comprehensive discussion of the technical aspects of crown-lengthening surgery must begin with enumeration of the various components of appropriate soft-tissue flap design.

Incision Design

INITIAL INCISION

Either an intrasulcular or subsulcular buccal incision is employed, which extends at least one tooth mesial and distal of the tooth to be crown lengthened. If an intrasulcular incision is utilized, a 15 blade is angled in such a manner as to remove the

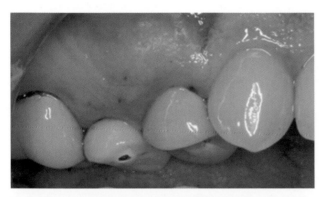

Fig. 2.25 A patient presents with final restorations on the maxillary first and second premolars. These restorations continue to dislodge. Note the incomplete passive eruption that is present.

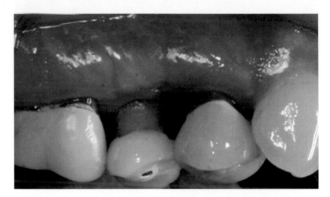

Fig. 2.27 Approximately 4 weeks post-therapy, the soft tissues have healed at the desired levels.

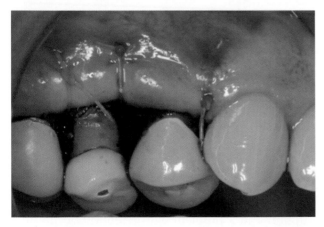

Fig. 2.26 Following crown-lengthening osseous surgery, adequate tooth structure is exposed for appropriate restorative intervention, and a more ideal gingival margin position has been attained. Note the unprepared enamel that was subgingival on the second premolar, due to the incomplete passive eruption that was present.

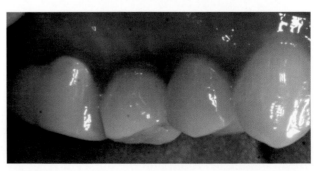

Fig. 2.28 Following final restoration, ideal, acceptable crown contours and gingival margin levels are evident. There were no retention problems with the final restorations.

sulcular epithelium. The incision is carried to osseous crest, with care being taken to scallop the buccal incision appropriately. In the case of a single-rooted tooth, the incision is scalloped so that long interproximal papillae are created. The buccal aspect of the incision mimics the ideal scallop of the buccal bone in health (Figs. 2.29, 2.30). As such, the slope and width of the scallop will vary from tooth to tooth. When an incision is made on the buccal aspect of a multirooted tooth, the incision is scalloped in such a way as to mimic the ideal scallop of the buccal alveolar bone, thus creating a "furcal papilla" (Figs. 2.31, 2.32).

If adequate keratinized tissue is present on the buccal aspects of the teeth to be treated, the initial incision is placed subsulcularly, taking care

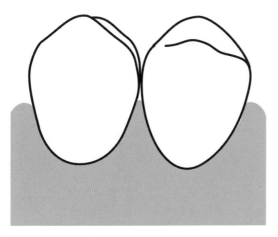

Fig. 2.29 A presurgical diagrammatic representation of a mandibular premolar area.

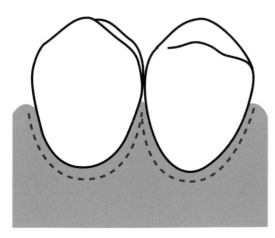

Fig. 2.30 The parabolae of the initial subsulcular incision mimic the contours of ideally scalloped buccal alveolar bone.

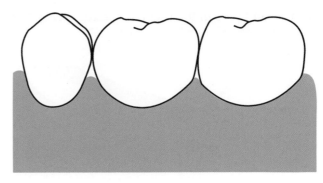

Fig. 2.31 A presurgical diagrammatic representation of a mandibular molar and premolar region.

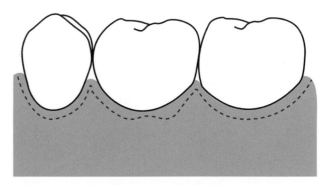

Fig. 2.32 Once again, the outline of the initial subsulcular incision mimics the ideal scallop of the buccal bone in health. Note the "double parabola" created in the furcation area.

to leave at least 3 mm of keratinized tissue between the incision and the mucogingival junction.

RELEASING INCISIONS

Mesial and distal releasing incisions are placed in such a manner as to ensure that the most mesial incision is placed on the distal aspect of the interproximal papilla, and the most distal incision is placed on the mesial aspect of the interproximal papilla (Fig. 2.33). The scalpel blade is angled so as to create a beveled incision, which will blend into the body of the papilla. A common technical error is to place the most mesial releasing incision on the mesial aspect of the papilla and/or the most distal releasing incision on the distal aspect of the interproximal papilla. In such a situation, the vertical releasing incision must be beveled into thinner buccal radicular soft tissues, rather than the thicker interproximal papilla. The net result will be more

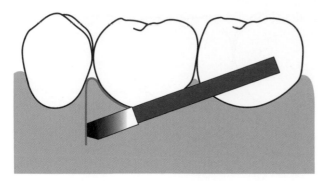

Fig. 2.33 The releasing incisions always bevel into the thicker tissues of the papilla, rather than the thinner buccal radicular tissues.

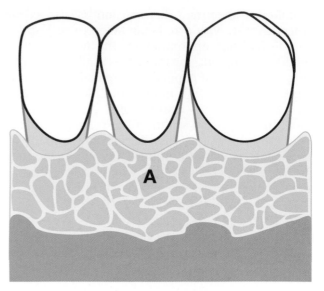

Fig. 2.35 Following the aforementioned sulcular and releasing incisions, a full thickness reflection is performed apical to the anticipated extent of osseous resective therapy. A = exposed alveolar bone.

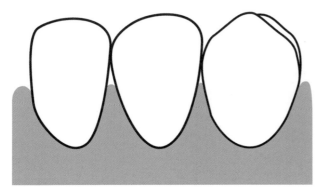

Fig. 2.34 A presurgical diagram of a mandibular cuspid and premolar region.

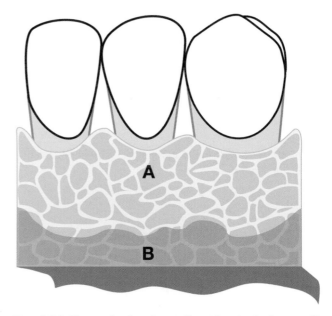

Fig. 2.36 Flap reflection is continued apically in a split-thickness manner, to afford retention of periosteal fibers and thus aid in flap repositioning and periosteal suturing. A = exposed alveolar bone; B = retained periosteum following split-thickness reflection.

postoperative scarring and greater evidence of the incision upon healing.

Vertical releasing incisions must be of adequate extension to allow repositioning of the buccal mucoperiosteal flap at the desired level following osseous resective therapy, as will be discussed.

The buccal flap is now reflected in a full thickness manner beyond both the mucogingival junction and the level of expected osseous recontouring. Reflection of the most apical few millimeters of the buccal mucoperiosteal flap is carried out in a split thickness manner, utilizing a 15 blade. Retention of periosteum over the apical bone will facilitate apical repositioning of the buccal flap, and flap retention in this position following suturing (Figs. 2.34 to 2.36).

A subsulcular palatal incision is made at such a level as to anticipate the final position of the osseous crest following crown-lengthening osseous surgery and bone recontouring. This crestally anticipated incision is scalloped in the same manner as already described for the buccal flap. Mesial and distal palatal vertical releasing incisions are placed, as previously described for the buccal mucoperiosteal flap design.

If the tooth to be crown lengthened is the terminal tooth in the arch, an internally beveled distal wedge procedure is performed. Buccal and palatal incisions are made on the distal aspects of the tooth (Figs. 2.37, 2.38). The incisions are beveled in such a manner as to undermine and thin the buccal and palatal tissues (Figs. 2.39,

2.40). The width between these incisions is determined by a combination of the amount of soft tissue to be removed and the expected reduction of buccal and/or palatal bony width during the crown-lengthening procedure. These "railroad track" incisions are carried beyond the tuberosity into the mucosal tissues distal to the terminal molar (Fig. 2.41). If the most terminal tooth present is a premolar, and it requires crown lengthening, these incisions are carried approximately 8–10 mm distal to the premolar.

Buccal and palatal vertical releasing incisions are placed as previously described, to facilitate flap reflection and debridement.

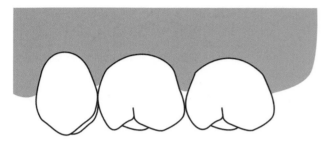

Fig. 2.37 A presurgical view of a maxillary molar and pre-molar region.

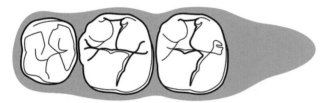

Fig. 2.38 An occlusal view of the same area demonstrating the distal wedge region.

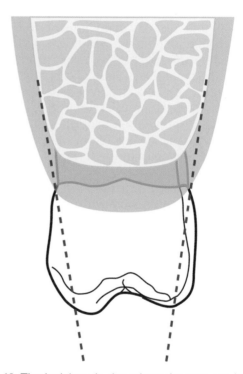

Fig. 2.40 The incisions in the tuberosity area are beveled so as to undermine and thin the buccal and palatal tissues distal to the second molar.

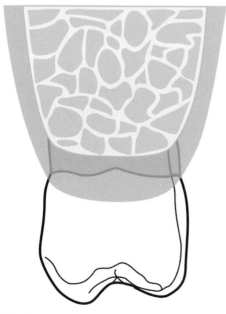

Fig. 2.39 A diagrammatic representation of a cross section of the tuberosity area distal to the second molar.

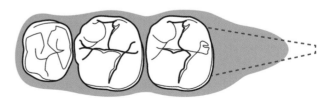

Fig. 2.41 The "railroad track" incisions are carried beyond the tuberosity into the mucosal tissue distal to the second molar.

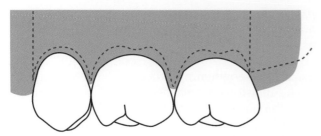

Fig. 2.42 A vertical releasing incision is placed on the distobuccal aspect of the second molar, to both provide greater visibility of the area and allow repositioning of the buccal flap independent of closure of the distal wedge region.

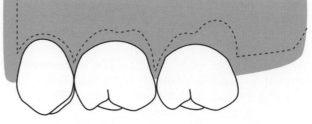

Fig. 2.43 If a distobuccal vertical releasing incision is not placed, an exaggerated scallop must be created on the distobuccal aspect of the second molar, so as to avoid soft-tissue repocketing following closure of the distal wedge area.

Even if a distal wedge procedure is to be performed, the aforementioned releasing incisions are placed on the mesial and distal aspects of the buccal and palatal flaps. Such an approach allows positioning of the buccal flap independent of the final soft-tissue position of the buccal distal wedge flap, as well as providing greater access and visualization for management of the distobuccal and distopalatal line angles of the terminal tooth in the arch (Fig. 2.42).

Failure to place a distobuccal vertical releasing incision in conjunction with performance of a distal wedge procedure leaves the treating clinician with two options : (1) an exaggerated submarginal scallop is employed as the incision rounds the buccal line angle of the most terminal molar, to allow suturing of the distal wedge soft-tissue flaps without unduly positioning the buccal flap more coronally than desired at the distobuccal line angle of the molar; or (2) the soft tissues are positioned in such a manner after suturing that soft-tissue repocketing will occur. A highly scalloped incision is not practical unless the patient presents with an exaggerated band of keratinized tissue on the distobuccal aspect of the molar in question (Fig. 2.43). Utilization of a distobuccal releasing incision to render closure of the distal wedge and positioning of the buccal flap independent of each other eliminates this concern.

The palatal flap is thinned, utilizing tissue forceps or a 1–2 pickup, to its most apical extent. This "internal wedge" of tissue is scored at its base with a 15 blade or Goldman-Fox 7 gingivectomy knife. The separated internal wedge of soft tissue is removed. If concomitant mucogingival therapy is required on the buccal aspects of the teeth being

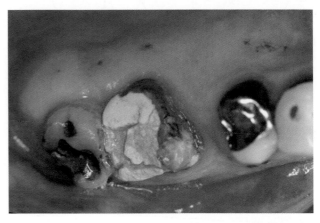

Fig. 2.44 A patient presents requiring crown-lengthening osseous surgery around the maxillary first molar.

treated, the internal distal wedge tissue will be employed as a connective tissue graft beneath a buccal flap. This technique will be discussed in Chapter 5.

The purpose of thinning the palatal flap is to ensure an even thickness of palatal tissues, which will conform to the created osseous contours upon suturing (Figs. 2.44, 2.45). Such thinning of the palatal flap helps ensure that a soft-tissue "ledge" will not be created on the palatal aspects of the treated teeth (Fig. 2.46). If a soft-tissue "ledge" did result following therapy, subsequent healing would lead to a more coronal final position of the palatal soft-tissue margin, a greater extent of palatal soft-tissue repocketing, and a compromised outcome to the crown-lengthening surgery. Soft tissues do not heal at sharp angles. Failure to manage soft-tissue morphologies during surgery has significant, undesirable posthealing ramifications.

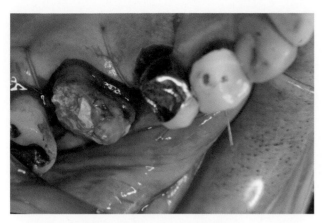

Fig. 2.45 Following appropriate flap design and osseous resection, the crestally anticipated palatal flap is sutured at osseous crest. Note the long papillae that have been created between the premolar and molar, so as to cover the alveolar bone as much as possible. Following healing, adequate tooth structure will be exposed for appropriate restorative intervention.

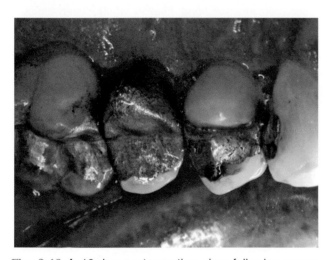

Fig. 2.46 A 10-day postoperative view following crown-lengthening osseous surgery demonstrates the ramifications of improper flap design. Note the palatal ledge of tissue, due to inadequate thinning of the palatal flap at the time of surgical therapy. As healing continues, the soft-tissue margin will develop more coronally than desired, resulting in a subgingival restorative margin and soft-tissue repocketing.

OSSEOUS RESECTIVE THERAPY

Osseous resective surgery is performed around the tooth to be crown lengthened, so as to obtain the endpoints previously described. A #8 round diamond bur is first utilized to reduce buccal and

palatal/lingual osseous ledging to the degree determined to be necessary to help ensure appropriate soft-tissue position and contour following healing (Figs. 2.47–2.49). In patients who present with a dense cortical plate of bone, a #8 round carbide bur is utilized under copious irrigation. It is important to realize that not all ledging and tori must be wholly eradicated. Rather, such bony protuberances must be reduced and contoured in such a manner as to allow the soft tissues to migrate over the established bony contours and heal in the desired manner and position. Osseous ledging may

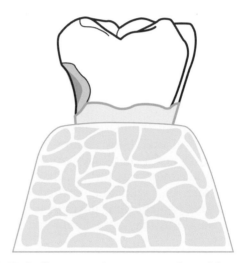

Fig. 2.47 A diagrammatic representation of buccal and lingual ledging, found following flap reflection.

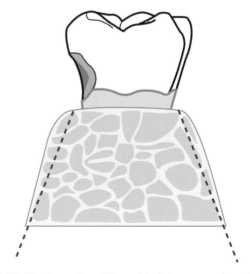

Fig. 2.48 The buccal and lingual ledging are reduced utilizing a #8 round diamond bur.

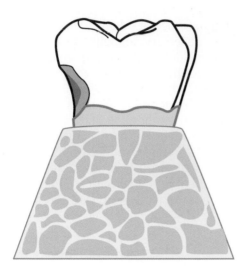

Fig. 2.49 A diagrammatic representation of the bone following reduction of the buccal and lingual ledging.

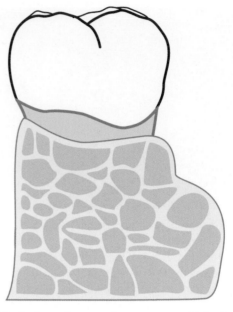

Fig. 2.50 A lingual torus is present, which does not approach the osseous crest, but will affect the final soft-tissue contours following healing of the overlying soft tissues.

need to be reduced to the marginal crest, or simply reduced away from the marginal crest, depending upon the preexisting bony contours. In similar fashion, tori do not usually have to be completely eliminated. Recontouring tori so that their bulk does not interfere with the desired soft-tissue migration and final healing position is all that is required. Bony tori may be encountered in one of four situations.

1. The first is the instance where the bony torus is in such a position as to play no role in either the ability to eliminate osseous defects or to influence soft-tissue healing. In such a situation, the torus is left untouched.
2. When the bony torus is in a position to have no influence on the ability to eliminate a bone crater or infrabony defect, but will influence soft-tissue healing, it should be reduced and sloped appropriately (Figs. 2.50–2.52).
3. In the third instance, the bony torus approximates the alveolar crest but does not mask an infrabony defect. In these cases, the bony torus is reduced significantly and essentially eliminated in its most crestal half. The bone is then contoured so that a gentle flow is obtained between the reduced crestal area of the bony torus and the more apical portion of the torus (Figs. 2.53–2.55).
4. Finally, a bony torus may be in position to either make up the buccal, lingual, or palatal wall of an infrabony defect, or to preclude

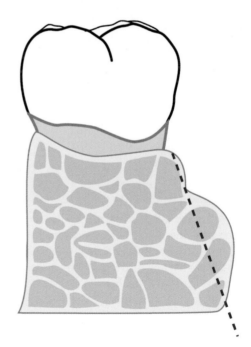

Fig. 2.51 The lingual torus is reduced.

elimination of this defect without treating the torus. In such a situation, the torus is completely resected in its most crestal half, and the contours are carried into a gentle slope

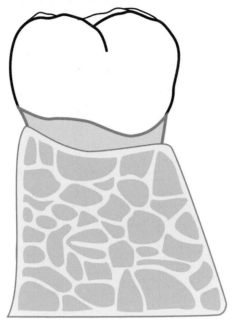

Fig. 2.52 Appropriate osseous contours are evident following reduction of the lingual torus of bone.

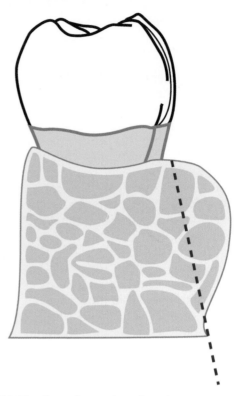

Fig. 2.54 The lingual torus is reduced.

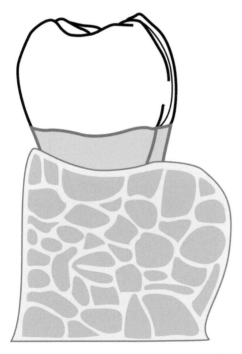

Fig. 2.53 A lingual torus is present which is confluent with the marginal alveolar bone. Failure to reduce this torus will result in soft-tissue healing in a more coronal position than desired, and subsequent repocketing.

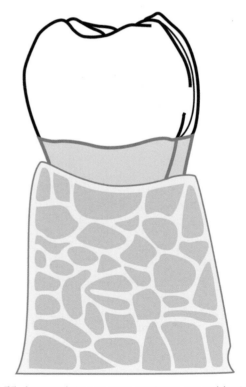

Fig. 2.55 Appropriate osseous contours are evident following reduction of the lingual torus of bone.

to be confluent with the more apical half of the torus (Figs. 2.56–2.58).

Reduction of osseous ledging and/or tori is accomplished within the context of developing desired osseous contours and "positive architecture." Failure to do so will result in repocketing, and a nonideal treatment result (Figs. 2.59–2.65).

The principles of osseous resective therapy have been well elucidated in the past. These principles include:

- Elimination and/or reshaping of osseous ledging and/or tori to such an extent that the bony contours will not hinder the development of ideal soft-tissue form following healing.
- Elimination of all interproximal osseous defects through resection, regeneration, or a combination of the two.
- Establishment of positive architecture, defined as development of appropriate parabolae on the buccal and lingual/palatal aspects of the roots, so that the bases of the parabolae are apical to the interproximal bone heights.
- Elimination of furcation involvements: This topic will be discussed in detail in Chapter 3.

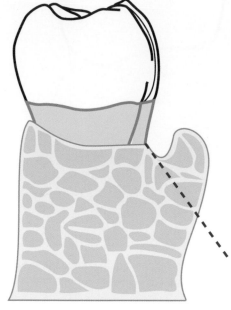

Fig. 2.57 The lingual torus is reshaped in such as manner as to eliminate the lingual component of the osseous defect.

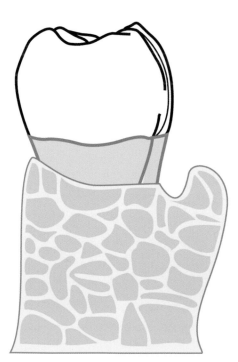

Fig. 2.56 A lingual torus is present, which is confluent with an osseous defect.

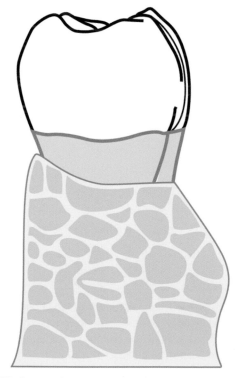

Fig. 2.58 Appropriate osseous contours are evident following reduction of the lingual torus of bone.

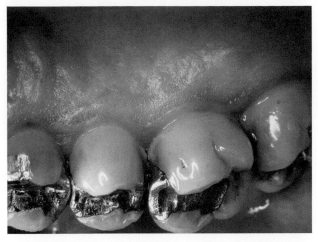

Fig. 2.59 A patient presents with 5–6-mm interproximal pockets, subgingival interproximal restorations, and bleeding upon probing. A palatal view demonstrates a "bulge" in the soft tissues between the first and second molar.

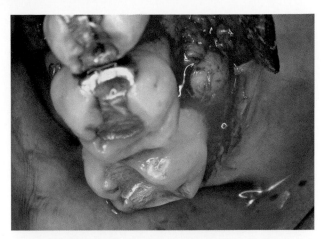

Fig. 2.60 Flap reflection reveals a palatal torus. This torus is in such a position as to render appropriate osseous therapy impractical without its elimination.

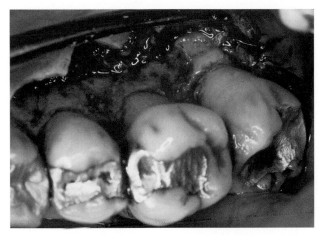

Fig. 2.61 The palatal torus is eliminated and ideal osseous contours are attained. Following suturing of the mucoperiosteal flaps at the appropriate positions, the resultant attachment apparatus and minimal probing depths will be highly maintainable by the patient.

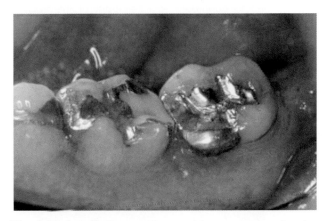

Fig. 2.62 A patient presents requiring crown-lengthening osseous surgery around the mandibular second molar.

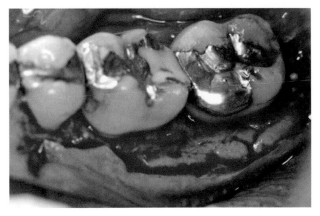

Fig. 2.63 Flap reflection reveals a significant lingual bony torus. If this torus is not reduced appropriately, the soft tissues will heal in a position more coronal than desired.

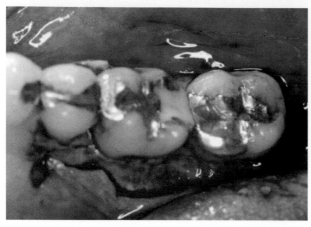

Fig. 2.64 The mandibular torus has been reduced and reshaped to both anticipate and participate in soft-tissue healing, and to contribute to attainment of the desired postoperative tissue contours.

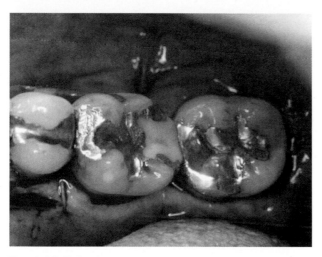

Fig. 2.65 Following suturing, it is evident that the soft tissues will heal at the desired levels.

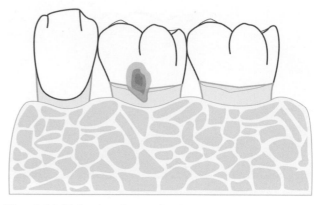

Fig. 2.66 Following flap reflection, the position of the carious lesion with regard to the alveolar crest, and the need for crown-lengthening surgery, are evident.

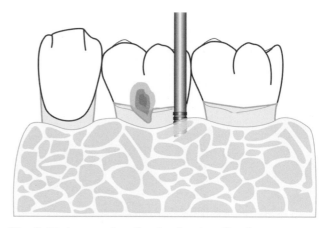

Fig. 2.67 A crown-lengthening bur is utilized to create an adequate dimension between the alveolar crest and the carious lesion on all aspects of the tooth.

A crown-lengthening bur is now employed in a circumferential manner around the tooth to be crown lengthened, ensuring that at least 4 mm of dimension is present between the planned final restorative margin position and the osseous crest (Figs. 2.66, 2.67). Any "moats" created by the crown-lengthening bur on the buccal or lingual/palatal aspects of the teeth are eliminated with the #8 round diamond bur (Figs. 2.68–2.70). If the tooth to be treated has not already been temporized for a full coverage restoration, thus limiting access to the mid-interproximal bone on the mesial and distal aspects of the tooth being crown length-

ened, the crown-lengthening bur is utilized as far interproximally as possible. A #2 round diamond bur is then employed to remove the small (approximately 1–1.5 mm in dimension) peak of bone which will remain at the mid-interproximal points of the tooth following utilization of the crown-lengthening bur.

If interproximal craters remain that are amenable to resective surgery, they are eliminated utilizing a #2 round diamond bur interproximally. The #8 round bur is once again employed to reduce any additional osseous ledging which has become evident as a result of preparing the "crown-lengthening trough" around the tooth to be crown lengthened. The osseous ledging is reduced on at least one tooth mesial and distal of the tooth to

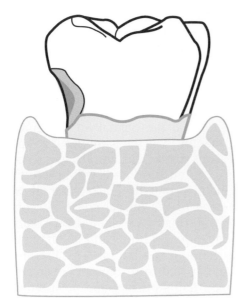

Fig. 2.68 A cross-sectional view demonstrates the osseous "moats" created by the crown-lengthening bur.

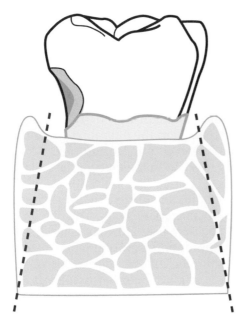

Fig. 2.69 The buccal and lingual alveolar bone are reshaped to eliminate the aforementioned osseous "moats."

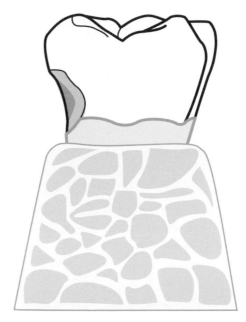

Fig. 2.70 Following appropriate osseous therapy, ideal contours have been attained and the desired biologic width has been established between the carious lesion and the alveolar crest.

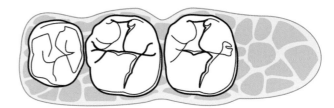

Fig. 2.71 An occlusal view demonstrates the buccal and palatal osseous ledging which is present at the distal aspect of the second molar.

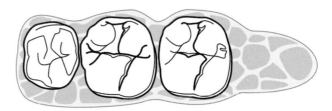

Fig. 2.72 The aforementioned ledging is reduced, to help control the contours and positions of the soft tissues following healing.

be crown lengthened. This is of paramount importance to help ensure a confluence of the hardtissue morphologies, and thus of the overlying soft tissues, upon healing.

Care must also be taken to reduce ledging that is present on the distobuccal aspect of the most terminal tooth, the distolingual/palatal aspect of the most terminal tooth, and on the body of the bone distal to the tooth in the area in which the distal wedge procedure has been performed (Figs. 2.71, 2.72). Failure to do so will result in significant

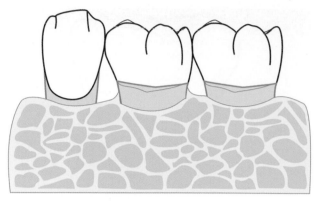

Fig. 2.73 A diagrammatic representation of the "widow's peaks" of bone, which are present interproximally following osseous resective therapy.

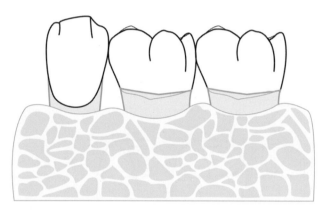

Fig. 2.74 The "widow's peaks" of bone are eliminated utilizing hand chisels.

soft-tissue repocketing and a soft-tissue level coronal to that desired upon final healing.

Ochenbein and Wiedelstadt chisels are employed to eliminate any widow's peaks of bone that remain at the line angles of the buccal and/or palatal/lingual aspects of the treated teeth, or interproximally (Figs. 2.73, 2.74).

The slopes of the created buccal and palatal/lingual parabolae are determined by both the morphologies of the roots in question and their buccal prominences. Teeth that are broader mesiodistally will demonstrate gentler parabolae with lesser slopes than their narrower counterparts. In addition, the more buccally prominent a tooth is in the arch, the greater the slope of the desired parabola. The same is true on the lingual/palatal aspects of the tooth in question. Patient biotype also plays a significant role in alveolar crest parab-

ola form. Patients with thinner, more highly scalloped biotypes demonstrate more pronounced parabolae than patients with thicker, less scalloped biotypes.

The buccal and palatal/lingual mucoperiosteal flaps are replaced and examined. If necessary, the crestal aspects of the flaps are recontoured so as to ensure that the palatal/lingual mucoperiosteal flap margin is at the same level as the established osseous crests. The buccal flap is recontoured if necessary to ensure that it will be positioned in such a manner that its crestal margin is at the attained level of the buccal crestal alveolar bone following suturing. Care should be taken not to remove any more keratinized tissue than necessary when retrimming the buccal flap. Retrimming of the palatal flap to ensure appropriate crestal anticipation upon flap suturing, and positioning of the buccal flap at the newly established alveolar crest level, are crucial steps in minimizing postoperative soft-tissue probing depths following osseous surgery. Neither insufficient flap reflection nor inadequate suturing techniques should be used as a rationale for overtrimming the buccal mucoperiosteal flap and removing keratinized tissues that are otherwise necessary for establishment of an adequate band of attached keratinized tissue. Rather, the clinician should reexamine incision designs and extend flap reflection in a split thickness manner if necessary, to afford the ability to passively reposition the buccal mucoperiosteal flap at the desired level, prior to suturing. If sutures are necessary to position the mucoperiosteal flap at the desired level, then flap reflection is inadequate. Sutures should be utilized in a passive manner, securing a mucoperiosteal flap in an already attained position. The clinician must also become fluent in appropriate suturing techniques to allow ideal positioning of the buccal tissues without excessive excision of needed tissues. It is usually more prudent to extend the buccal mesial and distal vertical releasing incisions, as well as the apical split thickness reflection of the flap to facilitate enhanced apical repositioning of the buccal mucoperiosteal flap than to remove needed keratinized tissue.

The buccal and palatal/lingual distal wedge soft tissue/flaps are reapproximated and examined. Depending upon the amount of osseous resection that was performed, one or both of these flaps may have to be trimmed at its crestal aspect. In addition, care should be taken to ensure that the flaps do not have to be further undermined and secondary wedges of tissue removed to ensure they conform intimately to the attained underlying bony contours following suturing. Inadequate thinning of the buccal and palatal/lingual flaps in the distal wedge area forces the tissue margins to "stand away" from the underlying bone excessively, and will result in greater soft-tissue repocketing following healing.

CLINICAL EXAMPLE FIVE

A patient presents with 5–8-mm interproximal probing depths, and 5–6-mm buccal and lingual probing depths, in the mandibular anterior region. Clinically, the tissues bleed upon gentle probing (Figs. 2.75, 2.76). Radiographically, significant osseous loss is present throughout this area of the patient's mouth (Fig. 2.77). Flap reflection reveals significant buccal osseous ledging, which

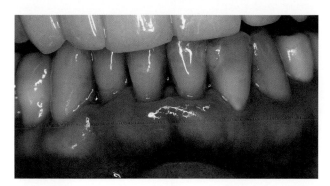

Fig. 2.75 A patient presents with inflamed, nonideal soft-tissue contours, probing depths of 5–8 mm, and bleeding upon probing in the mandibular anterior region.

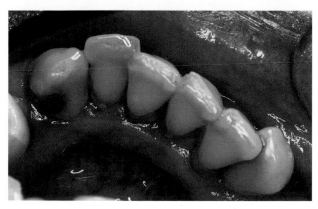

Fig. 2.76 A lingual view of the area.

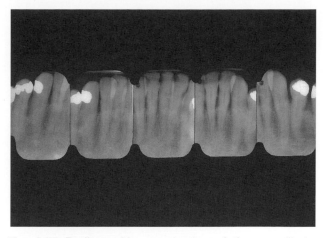

Fig. 2.77 Radiographic examination of the mandibular anterior region demonstrates significant osseous loss throughout the area.

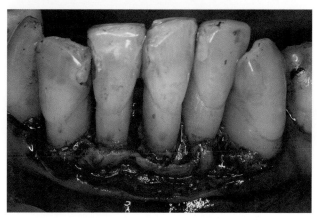

Fig. 2.78 Flap reflection reveals significant buccal osseous ledging, which is contributing to the development of moatlike buccal osseous defects.

makes up the wall of a buccal moatlike infrabony defect (Fig. 2.78). Lingual osseous defects are also evident upon flap reflection (Fig. 2.79). Osseous resective therapy is carried out on the buccal and lingual aspects of the teeth to eliminate ledging and the aforementioned moatlike infrabony defects. Osseous therapy is then carried out interproximally to eliminate all interproximal cratering (Figs. 2.80, 2.81). The buccal and lingual mucoperiosteal flaps are sutured at osseous crest with interrupted 4-0 silk sutures (Figs. 2.82, 2.83). Such a suturing material would not be employed today. One-week postoperative buccal and lingual views demonstrate excellent early healing and the

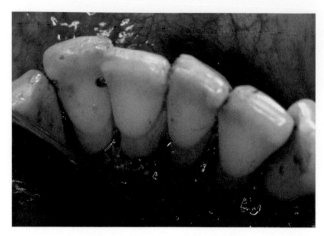

Fig. 2.79 A lingual view demonstrates lingual osseous ledging and infrabony defect formation.

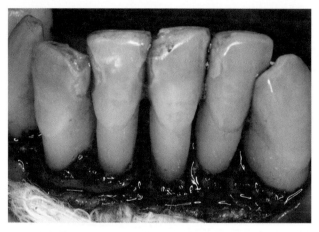

Fig. 2.80 Following osseous resective therapy, all ledging has been eliminated or reduced; and buccal, lingual, and interproximal defects have been eliminated.

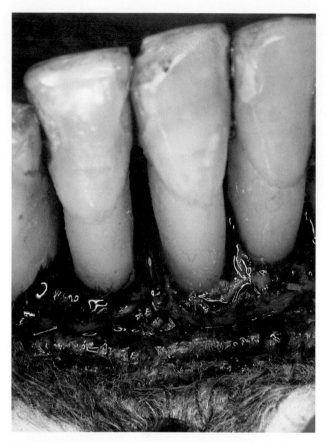

Fig. 2.81 A close-up of the mandibular anterior region following osseous resective therapy. Note the elimination of osseous ledging and all osseous defects.

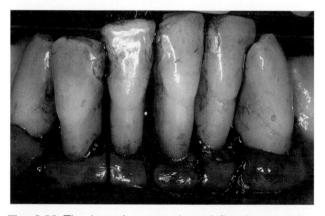

Fig. 2.82 The buccal mucoperiosteal flap is sutured at osseous crest with interrupted 4-0 silk sutures.

beginning of development of the desired soft-tissue contours (Figs. 2.84, 2.85). Following completion of soft-tissue healing, the patient will be left with probing depths of 3 mm or less around all treated teeth, and an attachment apparatus characterized by connective tissue insertion into the root surface, and a short junctional epithelial adhesion. Such an attachment apparatus is highly maintainable.

It is also important to ensure the necessary communication between the periodontist and the restorative dentist. Establishment of appropriate biologic width in an apico-occlusal dimension must take into account the preparation form to be utilized on each individual surface of a given tooth. For example, if 3–4 mm of exposed tooth structure is established between the alveolar crest and the anticipated restorative margin, and the restorative

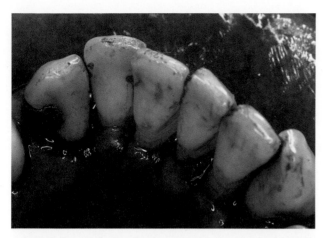

Fig. 2.83 The lingual mucoperiosteal flap is sutured after appropriate crestal anticipation, so that the soft-tissue margins are confluent with the established alveolar crest level.

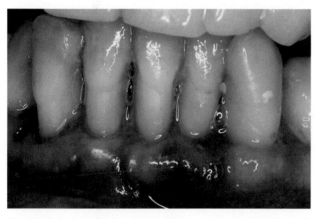

Fig. 2.84 A 1-week buccal postoperative view of the soft-tissue healing. Note the beginning of establishment of desired soft-tissue contours.

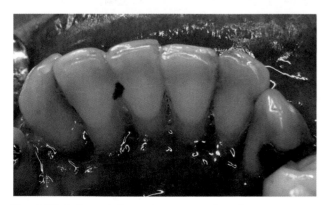

Fig. 2.85 A 1-week lingual postoperative view.

dentist is going to finish the preparation in this area with a long bevel, such a bevel will impinge upon the surgically established dimension for biologic width.

An in-depth discussion of tooth preparation designs following periodontal therapy will be undertaken in Chapter 6.

RAMPED OSSEOUS RESECTION

When the interproximal osseous morphology encountered is such that elimination of an interproximal crater through conventional techniques will result in either unacceptable aesthetic compromise in an aesthetically significant area, or will unduly remove supporting bone from around the teeth being treated, a modified osseous resective approach is utilized, as described by Ochenbein.

For example, due to the lingual angulation of the mandibular posterior teeth, interproximal osseous craters in these areas are often encountered that are deeper on their lingual aspects than on their buccal aspects. By removing the lingual wall of an osseous crater, carrying the appropriate positive osseous contours onto the lingual aspects of the teeth adjacent to the treated interproximal area, and keeping the buccal peak of bone intact or only slightly recontoured, a lesser degree of supporting bone and attachment apparatus is removed from the two teeth bordering the interproximal crater than would be the case employing conventional osseous resective approaches.

CLINICAL EXAMPLE SIX

A patient presents with 6–8-mm pocket depths between the mandibular left cuspid and first and second premolars. Clinical and lingual views demonstrate the nonideal soft-tissue contours and the inflamed nature of the interproximal tissues (Figs. 2.86, 2.87). Following flap reflection, significant osseous defects are present, as are buccal and lingual osseous ledging. The defects include an infrabony defect on the distal aspect of the cuspid, and a two-walled defect between the premolars which is confluent with lingual moatlike defects around the premolars (Figs. 2.88, 2.89). Conventional osseous resective therapy would result in removal of such significant amounts of osseous support that the long-term prognoses of the teeth might be compromised. However, careful examination of the morphologies of the osseous

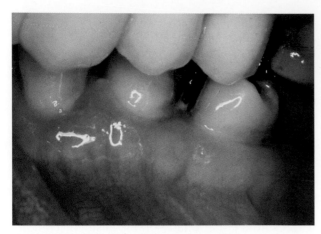

Fig. 2.86 A patient presents with significant interproximal buccal and lingual pocket depths. Note the inflamed nature of the soft tissues and the nonideal contours.

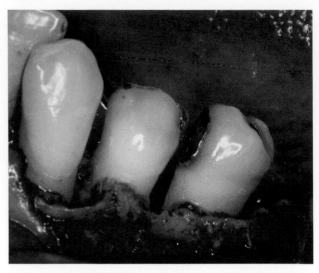

Fig. 2.88 Following flap reflection, significant osseous defects are present on the cuspid and premolars.

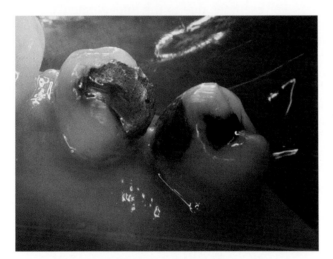

Fig. 2.87 A preoperative lingual view of the site.

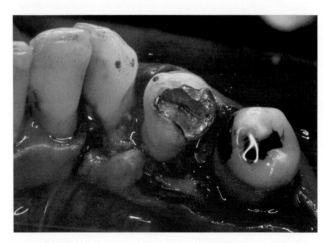

Fig. 2.89 A lingual view demonstrates the osseous ledging that is present, as well as the confluence of the osseous defect between the premolars with lingual moatlike osseous defects.

defects demonstrates that the defect between the cuspid and first premolar has an intact lingual peak of bone, and the defect between the two premolars has an intact buccal peak of bone. Therefore, osseous resective therapy is carried out as follows:

The buccal and lingual ledging are first reduced, thus eliminating the moatlike component to the infrabony defect on the buccal aspect of the cuspid. The interproximal bone between the cuspid and the premolar is ramped from the lingual to the buccal, maintaining the lingual peak of bone. The interproximal bone between the premolars is ramped from the buccal to the lingual, maintaining the buccal peak of bone. Ochenbein chisels are then utilized on the buccal and lingual aspects of

the teeth, to establish parabolae at the appropriate positions.

Following such therapy, all osseous defect have been eliminated and the maximum amount of bone support has been maintained around the teeth (Fig. 2.90). The flaps are now sutured at osseous crest following appropriate crestal antici-pation of the lingual flap (Fig. 2.91). Buccal and lingual 7-day postoperative views demonstrate excellent healing and the beginning of establish-ment of the desired soft-tissue contours (Figs. 2.92,

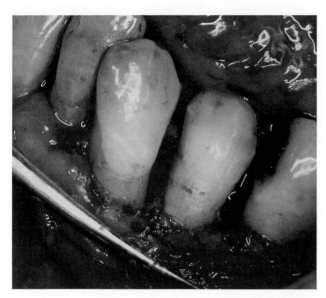

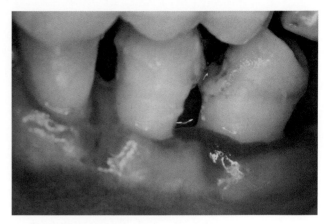

Fig. 2.92 A buccal 7-day postoperative view demonstrates excellent early healing and the beginning of establishment of the desired soft-tissue contours.

Fig. 2.90 Following osseous resective therapy including reduction of buccal and lingual ledging, ramping of the osseous defect between the cuspid and premolar toward the buccal to preserve the lingual peak of bone, ramping of the osseous defect between the premolars toward the lingual to preserve the buccal peak of bone, and establishment of appropriate parabolae, all osseous defects have been eliminated, while preserving the maximum amount of osseous support around the teeth.

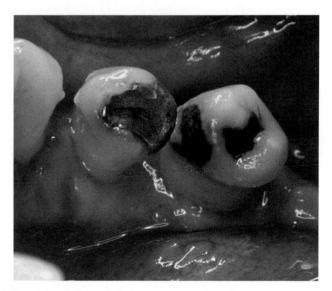

Fig. 2.93 A lingual 7-day postoperative view.

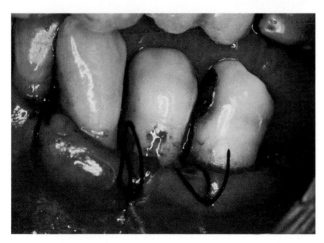

Fig. 2.91 The buccal flap is sutured at osseous crest. The lingual flap is crestally anticipated and sutured at osseous crest.

2.93). Following healing, the patient will be left with no probing depths in excess of 3 mm around the treated teeth, and a highly maintainable periodontal milieu.

In addition, utilization of such a technique in the maxillary anterior region to remove the palatal aspect of the interproximal crater while leaving the buccal peak of bone intact significantly ameliorates the aesthetic concerns commonly encountered when performing periodontal therapy in the maxillary anterior region.

Upon flap reflection, osseous resective therapy is carried out to provide a minimum of 4 mm of exposed tooth structure from the osseous crest to the planned restorative margin. This dimension allows for the development of an ideal attachment apparatus and approximately a 1–2 mm gingival sulcus. Following osseous resection, the mucoperiosteal flaps are sutured at osseous crest to ensure development of a predictable attachment apparatus. Studies have demonstrated that such therapy results in the establishment of the desired attachment apparatus of approximately 1 mm of connective tissue attachment crestal to the alveolar bone, followed by approximately 1 mm of junctional epithelial adhesion, followed by a 1–2-mm gingival sulcus supracrestally, upon healing. A gingivectomy type of surgical approach should not be utilized in these situations, as this modality would not address the spatial problem between the restorative margin and the osseous crest, resulting in a compromised attachment apparatus postsurgically.

Crown-lengthening osseous surgery is also utilized to remove redundant soft tissues, and to increase clinical crown length of short abutments, thus improving prosthetic retention.

Such an approach eliminates the potential problem of deep subgingival restorative margins when the clinician encounters subgingival carious lesions. As has been discussed, the most accurate of margins will trap plaque microscopically, resulting in gingival inflammation and an increased incidence of recurrent caries at the restorative margin-tooth interface. This scenario is further complicated as the marginal position extends subgingivally, and flutings and/or furcations are encountered on various teeth, rendering proper subgingival contouring of restorations impractical. When the added problem of operator visibility and isolation of the preparation is factored in, the situation becomes even less tenable. To assume that such a milieu is conducive to a healthy, predictable, long-term prognosis is to ignore both biologic concepts and clinical evidence.

CONCOMITANT BONE REGENERATION THERAPY

If bone regeneration is to be effected at the time of crown-lengthening osseous surgery, regenerative materials are placed after osseous resection has been carried out, prior to flap replacement and suturing.

While there is no doubt that the ability to regenerate damaged bone and attachment apparatus around periodontally affected teeth has greatly improved in predictability over the past few decades, the results of such therapy are far from

guaranteed. If regenerative therapy is to be employed, care should be taken to reduce the infrabony and/or furcation defect in which regeneration will occur to its most predictable state. Infrabony defects should be reduced if at all possible to a three-walled contained morphology. Class II furcation involvements should be reduced to such an extent as would be employed to eliminate a Class I furcation involvement in their horizontal depth through odontoplasty, as will be discussed in Chapter 3.

In addition, the clinician must realize periodontal regeneration will not occur, and regenerated tissues will not remain stable, if already enumerated periodontal treatment endpoints are not attained. Attempts to perform regenerative therapy in an area where restorative intervention is necessary and where the biologic width will be inadequate serve no long-term purpose, as periodontal inflammation will be reinitiated and breakdown of regenerated bone and attachment apparatus will occur.

The various costs attendant with regenerative therapy must also be considered, as will be discussed in Chapter 6.

MANAGEMENT OF THE MESIODISTAL DIMENSION

Failure to manage the mesiodistal component of the embrasure space results in a nonmaintainable situation highly prone to further periodontal and restorative breakdown. Rather than considering the tooth and its surrounding tissues as independent entities, the triad of the tooth, the gingiva, and the osseous housing must be envisioned and treated comprehensively, if long-term predictability is to be attained. While treatment of the osseous structures, and thus the overlying gingiva, will solve many of the challenges encountered when dealing with the embrasure area, only by addressing the tooth as well will the clinician truly solve the puzzle of more complex interproximal spaces.

Inadequate embrasure space due to tooth position results in an environment that is not conducive to the placement of cleansable restorative dentistry. Placing restorations in such tight embrasure spaces creates inaccessible plaque traps. This increased plaque accumulation is especially harmful due to the makeup of the supporting bone and soft tissues in these areas. When root proximity problems exist, the thin interproximal bone is cortical and highly labile in nature (Fig. 2.94). This bony septum is more vulnerable to rapid resorption in the face of plaque than a thicker interproximal septum would be. In addition, the overlying soft tissues are often retractable and friable in nature, offering less of a barrier to the initiation of the inflammatory process. As a result, the clinician is now faced with an area that is difficult to clean and more susceptible to inflammatory breakdown than other sites. Add to this environment the demands placed upon the periodontium by restorative dentistry, and the rapid breakdown that occurs in the area is easily explained.

Such tooth position problems may be solved in a number of ways. In many cases, orthodontics is a viable option. Repositioning of the teeth

provides an embrasure space morphology more conducive to long-term health. However, such an approach may not always be practical, due to clinical considerations or the patient's unwillingness to add time and expense to the overall treatment plan.

During periodontal flap surgery, crown proximity problems may be lessened or eliminated through the use of odontoplasty procedures. Odontoplasty is performed to the osseous crest, thus ameliorating embrasure space deficiencies due not to root proximity problems, but rather to tilting of teeth. Odontoplasty is equally effective in the modification of an embrasure space by "straightening up" the emergence profile of the tooth, which is defined as the angle at which the tooth emerges from the supporting osseous structures.

CLINICAL EXAMPLE SEVEN

A patient presents with mesial tilting of the mandibular second molar due to decay (Fig. 2.95). Clinically, the interproximal col form between the two molars is concave and inflamed (Fig. 2.96). Following flap reflection, the crown proximity problem between the first and second molars is evident (Fig. 2.97). Odontoplasty is performed on the second molar, both to eliminate the crown proximity problem and to provide a straight emergence profile of the tooth out of the bone on the mesial aspect of the second molar (Fig. 2.98). The increased mesiodistal dimension of the embrasure space between the first and second molars following ondontoplasty is evident (Fig. 2.99). The

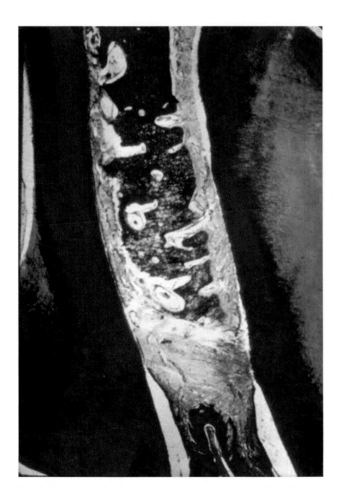

Fig. 2.94 A histologic specimen demonstrates the thin cortical, labile nature of the interproximal bone between the distobuccal root of a maxillary first molar and the mesiobuccal root of the maxillary second molar, when a root proximity problem exists.

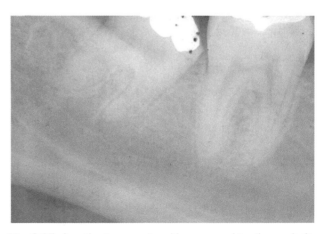

Fig. 2.95 A patient presents with a coronal tooth proximity problem due to a mandibular second molar having decayed and tilted mesially.

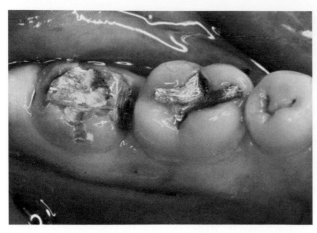

Fig. 2.96 The clinical view demonstrates the coronal proximity problem between the first and second molar, as well as the concave, inflamed nature of the interproximal soft-tissue col.

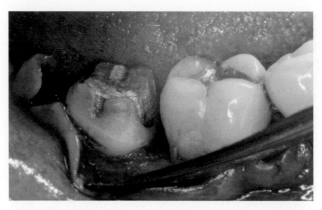

Fig. 2.98 Following crown-lengthening osseous surgery, odontoplasty is performed to "straighten up" the emergence profile of the tooth as it exits the bone on its mesial aspect, thus eliminating the coronal proximity problem between the two molars.

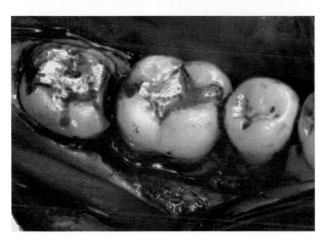

Fig. 2.97 Flap reflection demonstrates the inability to place a restoration on the second molar in a manner that will prove cleansable interproximally for the patient.

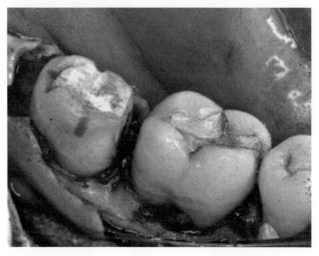

Fig. 2.99 Crown-lengthening osseous surgery and odontoplasty have resulted in elimination of the coronal proximity problem that was present. The odontoplasty that has been performed will now be carried over to the buccal and lingual aspects of the tooth to create a smooth confluence of the established tooth morphologies.

mesiobuccal and mesiolingual line angles of the second molar will now be recontoured to provide an appropriate confluence with the newly created mesial contours of the second molar.

The emergence profile has a direct influence on the morphology and quality of the surrounding soft tissues. The more acute the angle of the emergence profile becomes, the greater the soft-tissue "pileup," resulting in a decreased embrasure space dimension and hindrance of plaque control efforts. Such forces are at play when a redundant, retractable papilla develops on a mesially tilted molar, albeit on a smaller scale.

CLINICAL EXAMPLE EIGHT

The patient presents with a provisional restoration on the maxillary second premolar. Radiographically, a small infrabony defect is developing on the mesial aspect of this tooth (Fig. 2.100). A clinical view demonstrates inflamed interproximal soft tissues on the mesial aspect of the second premolar (Fig. 2.101). Following flap reflection, a nonideal

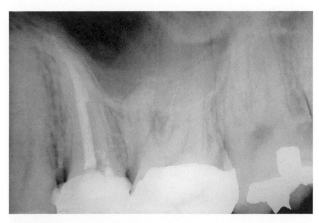

Fig. 2.100 A radiographic view of the temporized second premolar demonstrates the beginning of an early infrabony defect on its mesial aspect.

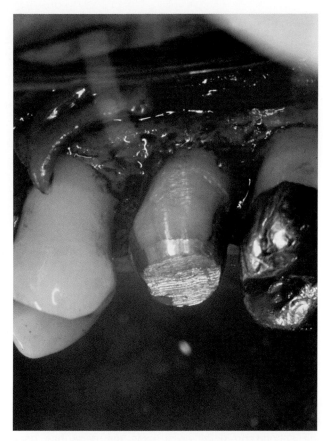

Fig. 2.102 Flap reflection demonstrates the nonideal emergence profile of the mesial aspect of the second premolar. This tooth morphology has resulted in soft-tissue pileup, plaque accumulation, and initiation of an early periodontal inflammatory lesion.

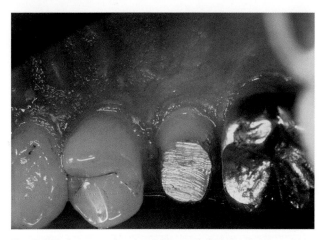

Fig. 2.101 Interproximal soft-tissue inflammation is evident on the mesial aspect of the second premolar.

emergence profile of the second premolar as it exits the bone is evident (Fig. 2.102). This emergence profile has resulted in soft-tissue pileup in the area, increased difficulty with plaque control, and the initiation of an early periodontal inflammatory lesion. Failure to appropriately manage this situation will result in a compromised prognosis after tooth restoration. Following appropriate osseous resective therapy to establish ideal bony contours, odontoplasty is carried out to the osseous crest to help ensure a more ideal emergence profile of the root out of the bone on all aspects of the tooth. Note the elimination of the "overhang" of tooth, which had been present on the mesial aspect of the premolar (Fig. 2.103). The buccal flap is sutured

at osseous crest and the lingual flap is sutured following crestal anticipation, as previously discussed (Fig. 2.104). An occlusal view demonstrates establishment of an ideal emergence profile of the tooth out of the bone (Fig. 2.105). Following healing and restoration, the patient will be left with a periodontal milieu which is conducive to appropriate home care efforts, and will help maximize the long-term health of the area.

Once again, it is crucial that proper communication exist between the periodontist and the restorative dentist when odontoplasty is performed. Following such a technique, the restorative dentist must not attempt to cover all cut tooth structure with his or her restoration. Such an approach would result in the restoration extending to osseous crest, as odontoplasty had been performed to this level. As previously discussed, impingement on

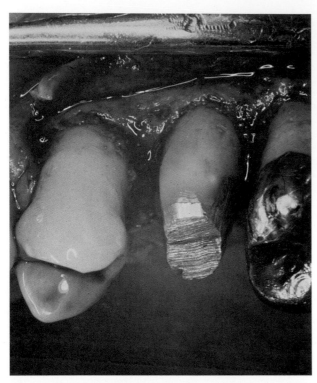

Fig. 2.103 Following appropriate osseous resective therapy and odontoplasty, adequate biologic width has been established and the emergence profile of the root of the second premolar as it exits the bone has been idealized.

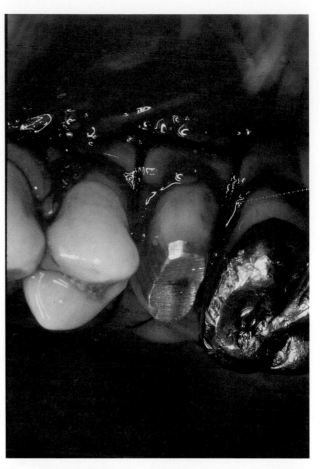

Fig. 2.104 The flaps are sutured at osseous crest, following crestal anticipation of the palatal flap.

biologic width creates an unstable, unhealthy situation.

Following 6 to 10 weeks of healing, tooth preparation is completed. The preparation should end either at the gingival crest, or intrasulcularly if necessary due to aesthetic concerns. The result will be a maximum of 1 mm of exposed cut dentin in a 1–2-mm sulcus, which is analogous to the clinical situation following root planing, and is easily maintained through proper plaque control efforts. The remaining 2 mm of cut tooth structure between the base of the sulcus and the crest of bone are protected by the connective tissue insertion and junctional epithelial adhesion of the post-surgical attachment apparatus.

MANAGEMENT OF THE BUCCOLINGUAL DIMENSION

Comprehensive periodontal and restorative management of the embrasure space also requires visualization of the buccolingual dimension. The extent

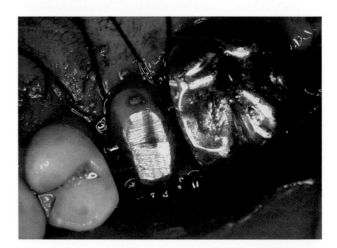

Fig. 2.105 An occlusal view demonstrates establishment of an ideal emergence profile of the second premolar as it exits the bone. Such an emergence profile will aid in patient home-care efforts and help maximize the long-term health of the area.

of buccal and/or lingual osseous ledging directly influences not only the buccolingual contours of the overlying soft tissues, but also the interproximal quantity and quality of these tissues.

To aid in this visualization, consider the pyramidal shape of the embrasure space (Fig. 2.106), where AB is the apico-occlusal dimension, EF is the mesiodistal dimension, and CD is the buccolingual dimension of the embrasure space. Point B is also the contact point between the two teeth bordering the embrasure space. The pyramid is broken into its component planes (Fig. 2.107), and is rotated 90 degrees (Fig. 2.108). As the extent of buccal ledging increases (AC), the angle of ACB must be more acute to end at the same point coronally. Therefore, in order for the soft tissues to pass under the contact point, they must migrate and heal at a more acute angle as the degree of buccal ledging increases. Soft tissues do not heal at such angles, but rather in a smoother, more confluent manner. As a result, as buccal ledging increases, the overlying soft tissues are often coronal to the contact point, and must pass underneath the contact point as they proceed toward the lingual aspect of the embrasure space. Such a scenario results in the development of a concave interproximal soft-tissue col form, with highly retractable buccal and lingual peaks (Fig. 2.109). This morphology is more conducive to plaque accumulation. In addition, when the interproximal soft

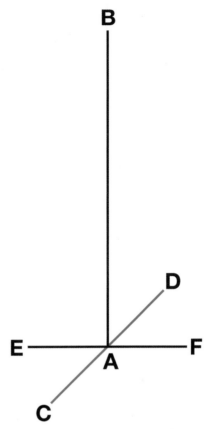

Fig. 2.107 The pyramid is broken into its three planes. A = alveolar crestal bone; B = contact points; C = buccal aspect of the interproximal alveolar bone; D = lingual/palatal aspect of the interproximal bone; E = mesial aspect of the tooth bordering the embrasure space; F = distal aspect of the tooth bordering the embrasure space.

tissues are in contact with the contact points of the teeth, they are nonkeratinized and thus more permeable to bacterial penetration (Figs. 2.110 to 2.113). Adding a restorative margin further complicates and exacerbates these problems. Fortunately, this concern is easily addressed at the time of preprosthetic periodontal surgery.

It is important to realize that the shape of the interproximal soft tissues is not a reflection of the morphology of the interproximal alveolar bone. Rather, the shape and keratinized or nonkeratinized nature of the interproximal soft-tissue col are influenced by the overall bony morphology, including the presence or absence of buccal and/ or lingual/palatal osseous ledging, and its relationship to the position of the contact point. When the interproximal soft tissues touch the contact point of the bordering teeth, the col form will be concave

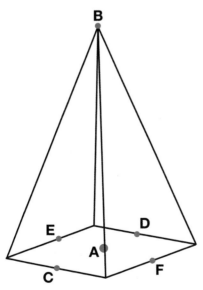

Fig. 2.106 To aid in discussion of the embrasure space, it is visualized as a pyramid.

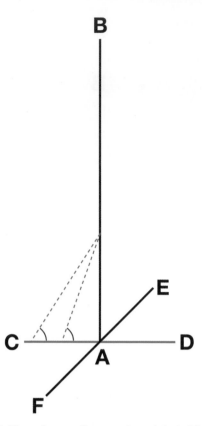

Fig. 2.108 The planar diagram is rotated 90 degrees. AC = the extent of buccal osseous ledging. The point established on axis AB is the contact point between the teeth. Note that the greater the buccal osseous ledging, the more acute angle the soft tissues must make when healing over the bony ledge to proceed to the lingual aspect of the embrasure space apical to the contact point. As soft tissues do not heal at acute angles, reduction of the buccal bone ledging must occur to help ensure that the soft tissues heal under the contact point, preventing formation of a concave, nonkeratinized soft-tissue col form.

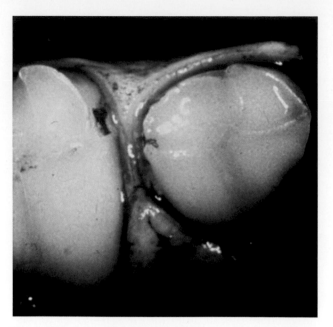

Fig. 2.109 A decalcified section demonstrates a concave interproximal soft-tissue col form. Note the retractable buccal and lingual soft-tissue peaks.

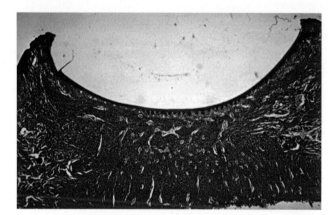

Fig. 2.110 When the soft tissues touch the contact point between the teeth, the overlying epithelium is nonkeratinized. The combination of a concave col form, nonkeratinized epithelium, and introduction of a restorative margin greatly increases the potential for periodontal breakdown.

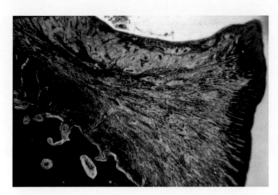

Fig. 2.111 Early stages of periodontal destruction are noted in the epithelium and overlying connective tissue fiber system of the interproximal col.

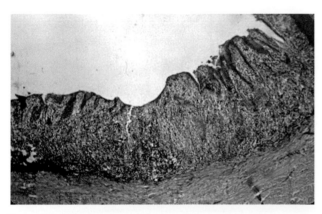

Fig. 2.112 Continued inflammatory destruction in the concave col form area has resulted in loss of epithelial integrity, and significant damage to the connective tissues in the region. Destruction of the supporting bone will now ensue.

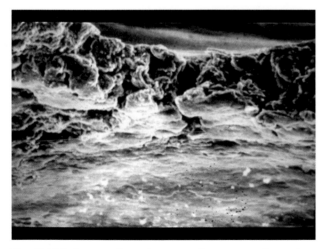

Fig. 2.113 A scanning electron microscope view of an ulcerated interproximal soft-tissue col.

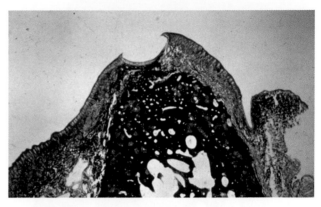

Fig. 2.114 Formation of a concave soft-tissue col form is not a reflection of the underlying interproximal bone morphology. Note the convex nature of the interproximal bony septum. However, because the interproximal soft tissues are in contact with the contact point between the two teeth, the col form is concave and nonkeratinized.

and the covering epithelium will be nonkeratinized. However, if appropriate osteoplasty is performed to allow the soft tissues to heal apical to the contact point, the col form will be convex and the covering epithelium will be keratinized (Figs. 2.114, 2.115).

Following flap reflection, osteoplasty and osseous resection are performed both to provide adequate apicoocclusal dimension for the establishment of the needed biologic width, and to reduce or eliminate buccopalatal/lingual ledging, thus producing a hard-tissue form more conducive to ideal soft-tissue healing (Figs. 2.116–2.118). By managing buccal and palatal/lingual ledging, and positioning the mucoperiosteal flaps at osseous crest during suturing, an environment is created that promotes healing of the soft tissues in a predictable, desirable, and cleansable manner. This reduction in buccal and palatal/lingual ledging allows the soft tissues to heal apical to the contact point, thus eliminating the concave, interproximal col form. In addition, when the interproximal soft tissues are not in contact with the contact points of the adjacent teeth, the soft tissues become keratinized and less easily penetrated by bacteria and bacterial byproducts. The net result is more cleansable, less vulnerable interproximal soft tissues.

CLINICAL EXAMPLE NINE

A patient presents with a subgingivally fractured mandibular first molar (Fig. 2.119). A decision

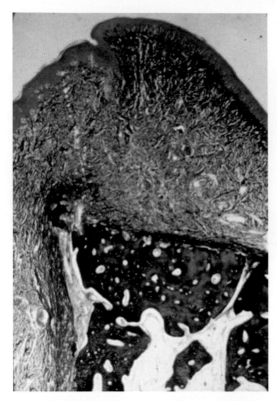

Fig. 2.115 Following appropriate osteoplasty to allow the interproximal soft tissues to heal apical to the contact point, the soft-tissue col form is convex, and the covering epithelium is keratinized. Such a situation is much more resistant to periodontal inflammatory breakdown than its concave, nonkeratinized counterpart.

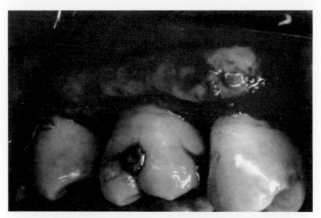

Fig. 2.117 Flap reflection demonstrates significant buccal osseous ledging. Failure to manage this osseous ledging would result in the soft tissues healing more coronally than desired, and the reinstitution of interproximal pocketing.

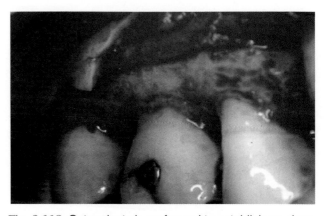

Fig. 2.118 Osteoplasty is performed to establish an alveolar morphology that is conducive to the soft tissues healing at the desired level, apical to the interproximal contact points.

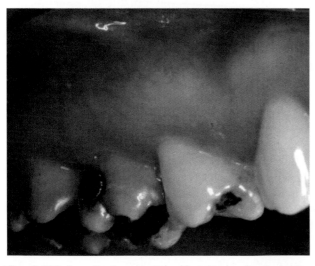

Fig. 2.116 A patient presents with interproximal probing depths of 5–6mm, bleeding upon gentle probing, and restorations that were subgingival interproximally.

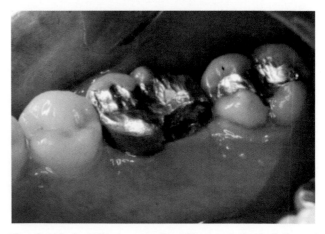

Fig. 2.119 A patient presents with a subgingival lingual fracture of the mandibular first molar.

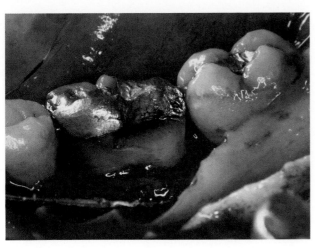

Fig. 2.120 Flap reflection demonstrates that the distolingual aspect of the tooth fracture is within 2 mm of the osseous crest. Therefore, utilization of a gingivectomy, electrosurgical, or laser approach would not afford an environment conducive to establishment of an ideal attachment apparatus post-therapy.

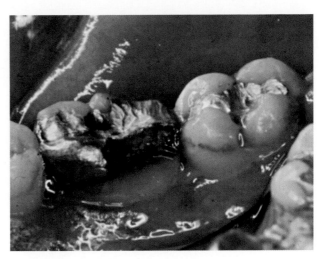

Fig. 2.121 Following crown-lengthening osseous surgery in all dimensions, adequate tooth structure is exposed for appropriate restorative intervention. Note the ideal soft-tissue form.

must be made as to how to treat this tooth. While it is tempting to perform a localized electrosurgical or laser procedure to eliminate adequate soft tissue to expose the tooth fracture and fabricate a restoration, such an approach will not be conducive to long-term health in the area. Flap reflection demonstrates that the tooth fracture is within 2 mm of the osseous crest on the distal lingual aspect of the tooth (Fig. 2.120). Therefore, failure to appropriately manage the tooth bone interface and establish ideal biologic width in all dimensions would result in a compromised attachment apparatus, and would increase the chances of development of a periodontal inflammatory lesion in the area. Osseous resective therapy was therefore carried out in all dimensions, as previously described, to establish appropriate biologic width and to create osseous contours conducive to participating in healing of the soft tissues at the desired levels and morphologies. Following healing, adequate tooth structure was exposed for appropriate restorative intervention, and the soft-tissue contours were ideal (Fig. 2.121). The tooth was subsequently restored utilizing a full coverage approach. A clinical view 26 years post-therapy demonstrates continuing periodontal and restorative health in the area (Fig. 2.122).

Failure to visualize and manage both the interproximal space and the tooth bone soft-tissue

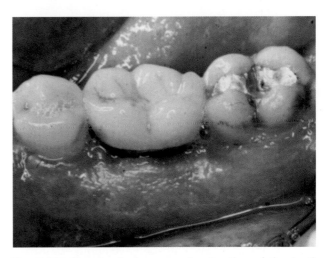

Fig. 2.122 Twenty-six years postrestoration of the tooth utilizing a full coverage approach, continued periodontal and restorative health are evident.

complex in a three-dimensional manner will result in a compromised treatment outcome.

CLINICAL EXAMPLE TEN

A patient presents with a provisional restoration on the lower first molar (Fig. 2.123). Following removal of the provisional restoration, the inflamed nature of the soft tissues and the need for crown-lengthening surgery are evident (Fig. 2.124). A

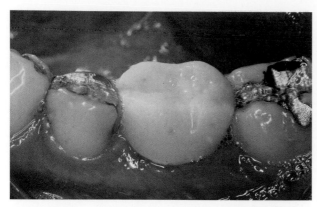

Fig. 2.123 A patient presents with a provisional restoration on the mandibular first molar.

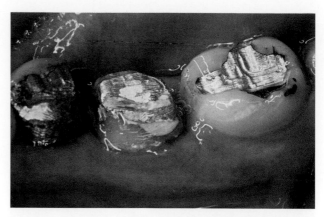

Fig. 2.125 A lingual view demonstrates the subgingival extension of the provisional restoration and the inflamed soft tissues in the area.

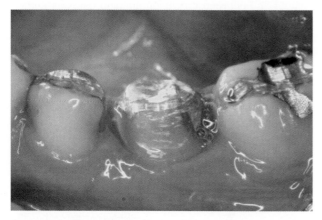

Fig. 2.124 Following removal of the provisional restoration, inflamed soft tissues and the need for crown-lengthening osseous surgery are evident.

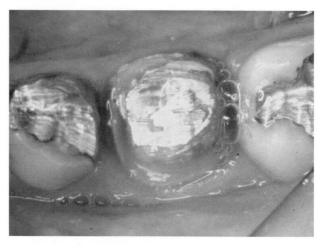

Fig. 2.126 Concave, nonkeratinized, inflamed interproximal col forms are present on the mesial and distal aspects of the first molar.

lingual view demonstrates the subgingival extension of the provisional restoration, and the inflamed tissues (Fig. 2.125). The concave, nonkeratinized, inflamed interproximal col forms on the mesial and distal aspects of the first molar are evident in an occlusal view (Fig. 2.126). Crown-lengthening osseous surgery is performed. However, the lingual ledging is not adequately reduced between the first and second molars. Following healing, a concave, nonkeratinized, inflamed interproximal col form is evident between the first and second molars, as a result of the soft tissues having to dip beneath the contact point as they pass from the lingual to the buccal aspects of the interproximal area (Fig. 2.127). Such a treatment result is nonideal and is directly attributable to insufficient osseous recontouring and a failure to treat the interproximal space as a three-dimensional entity.

Note that the soft-tissue col between the first molar and second premolar is convex and keratinized, and demonstrates no evidence of inflammation. This is the soft-tissue form and quality that should be expected following appropriately crown-lengthening osseous surgery.

CLINICAL EXAMPLE ELEVEN

A patient presents with a lingually fractured second molar (Fig. 2.128). Radiographically, bone and attachment levels around the tooth are excellent (Fig. 2.129). Flap reflection demonstrates the need to perform crown-lengthening osseous surgery

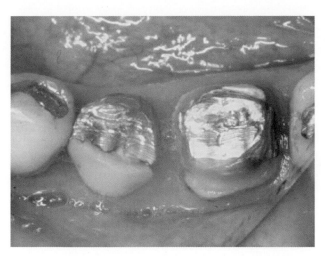

Fig. 2.127 Following crown-lengthening osseous surgery, the interproximal space between the first molar and second premolar is healthy and demonstrates a convex, keratinized col form. However, a concave, nonkeratinized inflamed soft-tissue col is present between the first and second molars, due to inadequate reduction of the lingual ledge of bone at the time of crown-lengthening osseous surgery.

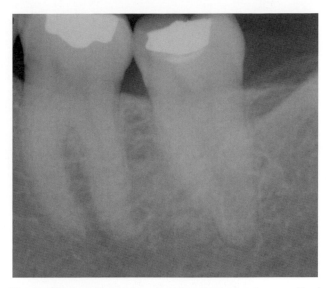

Fig. 2.129 A radiographic view demonstrates the excellent bone and attachment levels around the tooth in question.

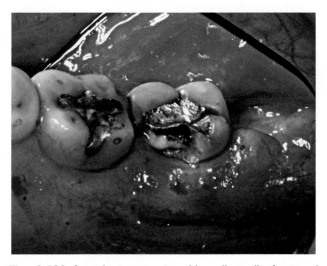

Fig. 2.128 A patient presents with a lingually fractured mandibular second molar.

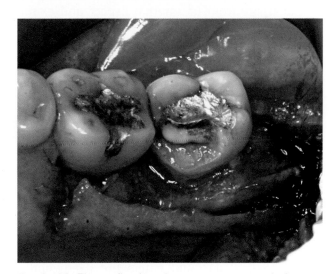

Fig. 2.130 Flap reflection demonstrates a tooth fracture within 2 mm of the osseous crest, as well as extensive lingual osseous ledging.

both apico-occlusally, to attain adequate dimension between the planned restorative margin and the bone crest, and buccolingually to eliminate lingual ledging and thus help control the final soft-tissue level and form (Fig. 2.130). Following appropriate crown-lengthening osseous surgery, healing and subsequent restoration, the area is healthy and stable both periodontally and restoratively (Fig. 2.131).

SUTURING TECHNIQUES

All mucoperiosteal flaps are sutured with interrupted, resorbable sutures. Ideally, a resorbable suture should be employed, which begins to lose its integrity 5–8 days post-therapy.

The assistant retracts the lip in such a manner as to apically reposition the buccal flap. The clinician passes the suture needle through the buccal flap at its most apical extent, engaging the retained periosteum. The suture needle is then

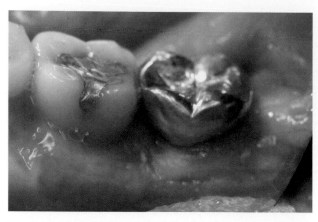

Fig. 2.131 Following crown-lengthening osseous surgery, healing, and subsequent restoration, the area is healthy periodontally and restoratively.

passed interproximally, and engages the palatal tissue in a vertical mattress approach, entering the palatal tissue from its internal aspect and exiting through its external aspect. The suture needle is passed back through the interproximal area. The assistant continues to apically position the buccal flap through appropriate cheek reflection. The suture is tied at the most apical extent of the buccal flap, utilizing a triple knot technique. The suture is flipped once around a Castro-Vejo instrument and the knot is tied. The suture is flipped a second time around the Castro-Vejo instrument and the knot is tied. The suture is flipped a third time around the Castro-Vejo instrument and the knot is tied. This procedure is carried out at each interproximal area.

The buccal vertical releasing incision is next sutured. The suture passes through the buccal mucoperiosteal flap and enters the fixed, nonreflected buccal tissues adjacent to the vertical releasing incision in a horizontal manner. The suture is tied in the manner described above. The vertical releasing incision is tied with a second suture, which is approximately at the crestal one-quarter mark of the vertical releasing incision, in a manner identical to that described for the suture at the more apical aspect of the vertical releasing incision.

If a distal wedge procedure has been performed, the distal wedge is closed with two interrupted sutures. The first suture passes through the external aspect of the buccal flap and through the internal aspect of the palatal/lingual flap, exiting at the palatal/lingual flap's external aspect, at the

points of the buccal and palatal/lingual distal wedge flaps that are closest to the tooth. The suture is tied in the manner previously described. A second suture is placed in an identical manner, near the most distal aspect of the distal wedge incisions.

INCOMPLETE PASSIVE ERUPTION

Patient presentation with a significant amount of the anatomic crown covered by soft tissues is often called incomplete (altered) passive eruption (IPE). It is important to realize that such a diagnosis may describe different clinical entities, requiring distinct therapeutic interventions.

While patients often present complaining of a "gummy" smile as a result of excess soft tissues covering varying portions of their clinical crowns, incomplete passive eruption (IPE) must not be considered only an esthetic concern. The redundant soft tissues coronal to the mucogingival junction do not attach to the tooth, as connective tissue attachment to enamel does not occur (Figs. 2.132, 2.133). Such a patient presents with pseudopocketing, which greatly increases the incidence of subgingival plaque accumulation and the chances of developing periodontal diseases (Figs. 2.134– 2.136). Therefore, IPE is a clinical entity that must be treated. Prior to embarking upon care, it is crucial that an appropriate diagnosis be carried out to differentiate between the two basic categories of IPE, as well as various contributing factors.

The patient must first be examined to determine whether the IPE is present only on the buccal aspects of the teeth, which is often the case, or on the palatal/lingual aspects of the teeth as well. A patient with IPE may present with the alveolar crests at least 2.5 mm apical to the cementoenamel junctions of the teeth in question, or with the alveolar crests within 2.5 mm of the cementoenamel junctions of the teeth to be treated. The relationship between the alveolar crests and the cementoenamel junctions is easily determined through a combination of radiographic examination and gentle bone sounding. In addition, the buccal and/or palatal/lingual osseous contours must be assessed, to determine whether or not buccal and or palatal/lingual osseous ledging are present. Such ledging often contributes to the coronal position of the soft tissues, and may dictate healing of the soft tissues in a more coronal position than desired. Finally, the apico-occlusal and

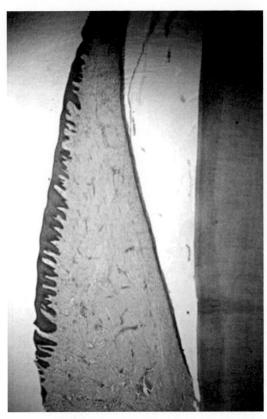

Fig. 2.132 A histologic specimen demonstrates the inability to attain connective tissue attachment to enamel. Note the long junctional epithelium, which is evident in the decalcified section.

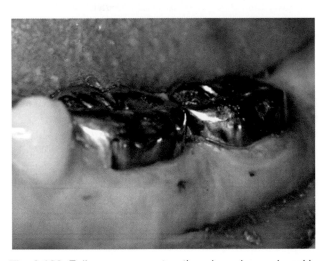

Fig. 2.133 Full-coverage restorations have been placed in the presence of incomplete passive eruption. The combination of soft-tissue pocketing and increased plaque accumulation at the restorative margin tooth interface has resulted in the initiation of soft-tissue inflammation. The outline of the inflammation is evident clinically.

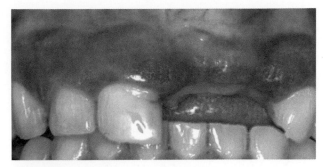

Fig. 2.134 A patient presents with incomplete passive eruption.

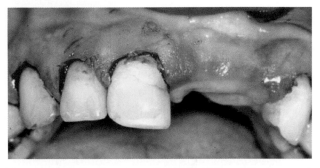

Fig. 2.135 Following recontouring of the redundant soft tissues, the increased plaque and calculus accumulation, which had occurred in the soft-tissue pockets, is evident.

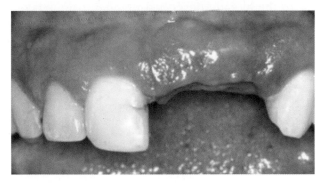

Fig. 2.136 Following healing, the soft tissues are at the desired levels, and the milieu is conducive to appropriate patient home-care efforts.

buccolingual dimensions of the attached and unattached keratinized soft tissues that are present must be assessed.

It is uncommon to encounter a patient with incomplete passive eruption and inadequacy in the buccolingual dimension of the buccal keratinized tissues. However, such a situation may be found in patients with a delicate, more highly scalloped biotype. In these cases, a connective tissue graft is placed beneath the buccal flap at the time of hard- and/or soft-tissue recontouring. Although rare, it is imperative to recognize this clinical scenario, so as to avoid postoperative aesthetic disaster. Failure to augment soft tissues which are thin buccolingually will result in a significant degree of soft-tissue resorption and recession following surgical insult, and a nonaesthetic final result.

If the osseous crests are at least 2.5 mm apical to the cementoenamel junctions of the teeth to be treated, no buccal osseous ledging is present, and adequate keratinized tissues are present to allow retention of at least 3 mm of attached keratinized tissue following soft-tissue recontouring to the desired level, the soft tissues may be recontoured without osseous resection, utilizing either a 15 blade or a laser (Figs. 2.137, 2.138).

If the osseous crests are at least 3 mm apical to the cementoenamel junctions of the teeth to be treated, if no buccal osseous ledging is present, and inadequate keratinized tissues are present to allow retention of at least 3 mm of attached keratinized tissue following soft-tissue recontouring to the desired level, therapy cannot be carried out through utilization of a laser, as such an approach would result in a potential mucogingival problem for the patient. In such a situation, flap reflection is carried out in the already described manner, care is taken to ensure that the osseous crests are 2.5 mm apical

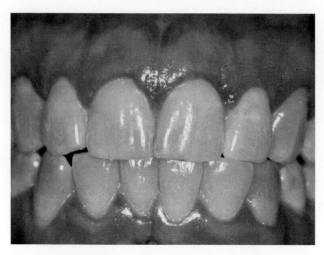

Fig. 2.138 Due to the aforementioned clinical scenario, soft-tissue recontouring is carried out without concomitant osseous resection. The final treatment outcome demonstrates soft-tissue healing at the desired levels with relation to the cementoenamel junctions of the teeth.

to the cementoenamel junctions of the teeth on their buccal and palatal/lingual aspects, and the mucoperiosteal flaps are sutured at the levels of the cementoenamel junctions, employing interrupted suturing techniques as previously described.

If the osseous crests are at least 2.5 mm apical to the cementoenamel junctions of the teeth to be treated, significant buccal and/or palatal ledging is present, and adequate buccal keratinized tissue is noted to allow retention of at least 3 mm of attached keratinized tissue following appropriate soft-tissue recontouring, a buccal mucoperiosteal flap is raised as follows:

A scalloped subsulcular incision is carried out at the desired final soft-tissue level. The scallops of the incision are identical to those previously discussed. Vertical releasing incisions are placed on the mesial and distal aspects of the mucoperiosteal flap, as previously discussed. Flap reflection and reduction of osseous ledging are carried out as already detailed. Finally, the flaps are sutured in a replaced manner with interrupted resorbable sutures.

If the osseous crests are at least 2.5 mm apical to the cementoenamel junctions of the teeth to be treated, significant osseous ledging is present, and adequate buccal attached keratinized tissues are not present to allow submarginal incision placement as previously described with retention of 3 mm of attached keratinized tissue, therapy proceeds as follows:

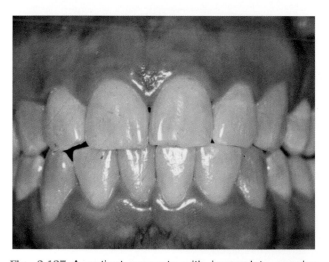

Fig. 2.137 A patient presents with incomplete passive eruption. A space of 2.5 mm is present between the crest of the alveolar bone and the cementoenamel junctions of the teeth, no buccal osseous ledging is present, and adequate keratinized tissue is evident.

A scalloped sulcular incision, with mesial and distal vertical releasing incisions, is carried out as previously described. Following flap reflection, osseous recontouring is carried out to reduce buccal and palatal/osseous lingual ledging to such an extent as to ensure final soft-tissue healing at the desired crestally anticipated bone levels on the palatal/lingual aspects of the teeth, and repositioned flap levels on the buccal aspects of the teeth. The flaps are sutured with interrupted, resorbable sutures.

If the osseous crests are within 3 mm of the cementoenamel junctions of the teeth to be treated, and adequate keratinized tissue is present to allow subsulcular incisions at the desired final soft-tissue level while still retaining at least 3 mm of attached keratinized tissue, therapy proceeds in one of the following manners:

If no buccal ledging is present, subsulcular incisions are made at the desired final soft-tissue levels. A specifically designed piezo surgical tip is then utilized to reshape and resect the alveolar crests to a position 2.5 mm apical to the cementoenamel junctions of the teeth. Following healing, all soft-tissue pocketing is eliminated, and the soft tissues are at the desired post-therapeutic levels to maximize aesthetic treatment outcomes.

CLINICAL EXAMPLE TWELVE

A 16-year-old patient presented having completed orthodontic therapy (Figs. 2.139–2.141). The

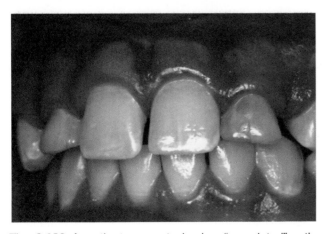

Fig. 2.139 A patient presents having "completed" orthodontic therapy, and bonding on the maxillary anterior teeth, in an attempt to close the postorthodontic diastemata. Four to five millimeters of soft-tissue probing are noted on the buccal aspects of the maxillary anterior teeth.

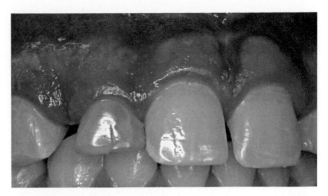

Fig. 2.140 A close-up demonstrates the residual diastemata and the bonding that has been placed. Note that inadequate bands of keratinized tissue are present to allow for subsulcular incisions to the desired final tissue level.

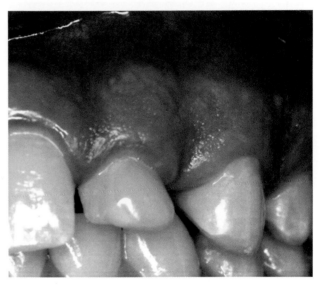

Fig. 2.141 A clinical view of the maxillary left anterior region demonstrates the bonding that has been placed in an effort to improve the patient's aesthetic profile.

patient was referred because she was unhappy with the "short appearance of her teeth." Her restorative dentist noted that there were 4–5 mm of soft-tissue pocketing around all maxillary anterior teeth. Bone sounding confirmed that the osseous crests were at least 2.5 mm apical to the cementoenamel junctions on all maxillary anterior teeth. However, adequate bands of keratinized tissue were not present to allow subsulcular incisions to the extent necessary, without compromising the amount of attached keratinized tissue that would be present postsurgically. Therefore, incisions were made that were approximately 1 mm subsulcular, and a buccal mucoperiosteal flap was reflected with releasing incisions, as previously described. Once care was taken to confirm that the alveolar crests were indeed at least 2.5 mm apical to the cementoenamel junctions of the teeth, the mucoperiosteal flaps were sutured at the levels of the cementoenamel junctions (Fig. 2.142). Eight weeks post-therapy, the soft tissues had healed at the desired levels (Fig. 2.143). Unfortunately, the diastemata still present following orthodontic therapy were now evident. In addition, it was obvious that the bonding the restorative dentist had placed in an attempt to close postorthodontic diastemata had not been placed along the long axes of the teeth

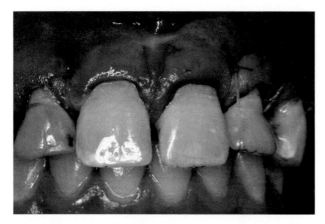

Fig. 2.142 Incisions were made 1 mm subsulcularly, a buccal mucoperiosteal flap was reflected, and care was taken to ascertain that the alveolar crests were at least 2.5 mm from the cementoenamel junctions of the teeth. The mucoperiosteal flap was then sutured at the desired final soft-tissue level utilizing interrupted gut sutures.

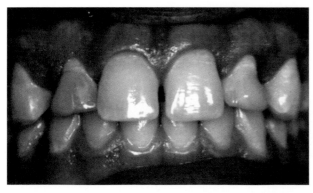

Fig. 2.143 Eight weeks post-therapy, the soft tissues have healed at the desired levels.

(Fig. 2.144). The patient will have to undergo additional orthodontic therapy to appropriately space the maxillary anterior teeth, followed by definitive restorative intervention (Fig. 2.145).

It is crucial that all incomplete passive eruption be treated, and the desired final soft-tissue

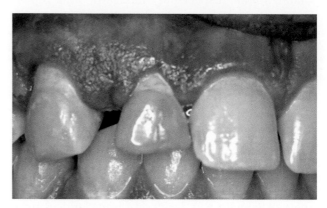

Fig. 2.144 Both the extent of the diastema between the lateral incisor and cuspid and the bonding that is in place are evident.

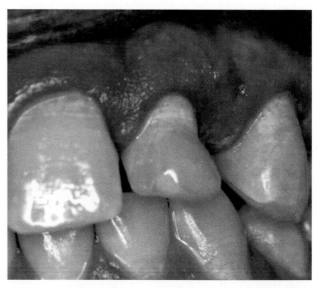

Fig. 2.145 The bonding that had previously been placed was not along the long axes of the teeth. In addition, the significant diastemata that are present resulted in patient dissatisfaction and the need for additional orthodontic therapy to better distribute the spacing between the teeth prior to definitive restorative intervention. Elimination of the incomplete passive eruption prior to completion of orthodontic therapy would have avoided the need for reinitiation of such care.

positions be established, prior to completion of orthodontic therapy. Failure to do so increases the chances of having to reinitiate orthodontic care, and often leads to patient dissatisfaction. By establishing the final hard and soft-tissue positions prior to completion of orthodontic therapy, the orthodontist is able to appropriately align teeth and ensure maximization of both functional and aesthetic treatment outcomes.

If osseous ledging is present, subsulcular incisions are carried out with mesial and distal vertical releasing incisions, as previously described. Split thickness flap reflection is accomplished. Osseous resective therapy is carried out to ensure a dimension of 2.5 mm between the osseous crests and the cementoenamel junctions of the teeth being treated. Osseous ledging is reduced as previously described when discussing crown-lengthening osseous surgery. An Ochenbein bone chisel is utilized to attain the desired bone contours. If no osseous ledging is present, no buccal bone reduction is carried out. The buccal mucoperiosteal flap is sutured in a replaced position utilizing interrupted, resorbable sutures.

CLINICAL EXAMPLE THIRTEEN

A patient presents with severe incomplete passive eruption, and anterior probing depths of 5–6 mm. More than adequate keratinized tissue is present to allow subsulcular incisions at the desired levels without compromising the amount of attached keratinized tissue that will be present post-therapy (Fig. 2.146). The alveolar crests are within 2.5 mm of the cementoenamel junctions (Fig. 2.147). A subsulcular incision is carried out on the maxillary left central incisor to the desired final soft-tissue

position (Fig. 2.148). Note the amount of soft tissue that has been removed, as compared to the untreated contra lateral central incisor. The tissue on the maxillary right central incisor has been recontoured to the desired level, and a periodontal probe in place demonstrates that the alveolar crest on the buccal aspect of the maxillary right lateral incisor is within 1.5 mm of the cementoenamel junction of the tooth (Fig. 2.149). Soft-tissue recontouring is completed across all maxillary anterior teeth (Fig. 2.150). A specifically designed piezo surgery tip is now employed to reshape and resect the alveolar crest to a distance 2.5 mm apical to the cementoenamel junctions of the teeth (Fig. 2.151). This therapy is performed on all teeth, as necessary. Approximately 8 weeks post-therapy, healing is uneventful, soft tissues are at the desired levels,

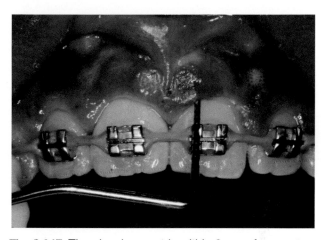

Fig. 2.147 The alveolar crest is within 2 mm of cementoenamel junction on the maxillary left central incisor. Such a relationship exists on all of the patient's maxillary anterior teeth.

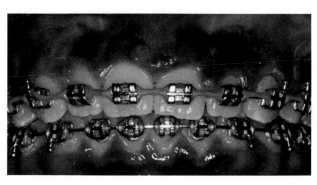

Fig. 2.146 A patient presents with incomplete passive eruption, and buccal probing depths of 5–6 mm.

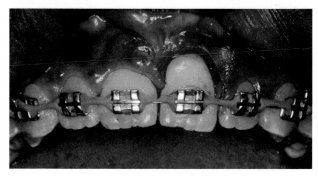

Fig. 2.148 The soft tissue has been recontoured to the desired level on the buccal aspect of the maxillary left central incisor.

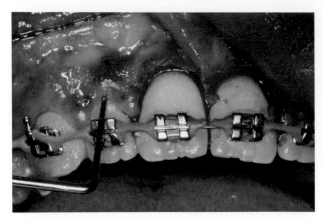

Fig. 2.149 Soft-tissue recontouring has been carried out on the buccal aspects of both maxillary incisors. Bone sounding demonstrates that the alveolar crest is within 1.5 mm of the cementoenamel junction of the maxillary right lateral incisor.

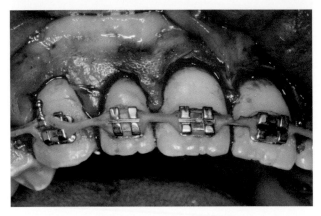

Fig. 2.150 Soft-tissue recontouring has been carried out to the desired levels on all maxillary anterior teeth.

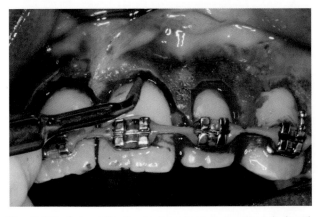

Fig. 2.151 A specifically designed piezo surgical tip is utilized to resect the alveolar crest to a distance 3 mm from the cementoenamel junctions of all maxillary anterior teeth.

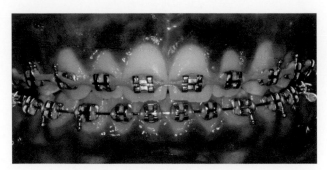

Fig. 2.152 Eight weeks post-therapy, the soft tissues have healed at the desired levels, all soft-tissue pocketing is eliminated, and the patient's aesthetic profile is improved.

and all soft-tissue pocketing has been eliminated (Fig. 2.152).

If the osseous crests are within 2.5 mm of the cementoenamel junctions of the teeth to be treated, and inadequate keratinized tissue is present to allow utilization of submarginal incisions to the desired final tissue level and still retain 3 mm of attached keratinized tissue, treatment is carried out as follows:

An intrasulcular incision is utilized as discussed for crown-lengthening osseous surgery. Incision scallop design, vertical releasing incisions, and partial thickness flap reflection are carried out as already described. If osseous ledging is present, it is reduced as previously described when discussing crown-lengthening osseous surgery. If no osseous ledging is present, no buccal bone reduction is carried out. Osseous resective therapy is carried out to ensure a dimension of 2.5 mm between the osseous crests and the cementoenamel junctions of the teeth being treated. An Ochenbein bone chisel is utilized to attain the desired bone contours. Following appropriate osseous resective therapy, the buccal flap is apically repositioned and sutured at the desired final soft-tissue level utilizing interrupted, resorbable sutures.

Note that in all the situations described above, the interproximal tissues are not removed. Rather, they are retained to help preserve interproximal papillae and maximize esthetic treatment outcomes. If these interproximal buccal soft tissues are not ideal in contour due to the IPE that is present, they are gently reshaped utilizing a 15 blade and an external incision approach, leaving the body of the interproximal soft-tissue papilla intact.

CLINICAL EXAMPLE FOURTEEN

A patient presents at the end stages of orthodontic therapy with severe incomplete passive eruption, and soft-tissue probing depths of 5–6 mm (Fig. 2.153). Flap reflection demonstrates that the alveolar crests are at the cementoenamel junctions of the teeth (Fig. 2.154). Failure to perform osseous resection and provide 2.5 mm of dimension between the alveolar crest and the cementoenamel junction would result in the soft tissues healing at a position more coronal than desired, and the reinitiation of soft-tissue pocketing. After appropriate osseous therapy has been carried out and the mucoperiosteal flap has been positioned at the desired level, healing is uneventful, resulting in improvement of the aesthetic profile and elimination of soft-tissue pocketing (Fig. 2.155).

CLINICAL EXAMPLE FIFTEEN

A patient presents with gingival disharmony, incomplete passive eruption, and periodontal pocketing of 5–6 mm in the anterior region (Fig. 2.156). A subsulcular buccal incision is made to the desired level of final soft-tissue healing (Fig. 2.157). Flap reflection reveals alveolar crests within 2 mm of the cementoenamel junctions of the maxillary anterior teeth, and significant buccal ledging (Fig. 2.158). Osseous resective therapy is carried

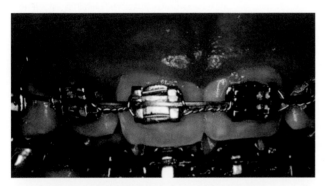

Fig. 2.153 A patient in the midst of orthodontic therapy presents with marked incomplete passive eruption.

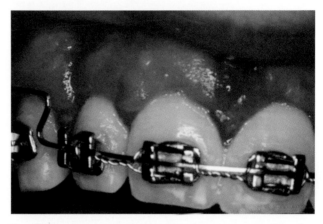

Fig. 2.155 Following appropriate osseous resection, flap positioning, and healing, the soft tissues are at the desired levels. Soft-tissue pocketing is eliminated, and the aesthetic profile is improved.

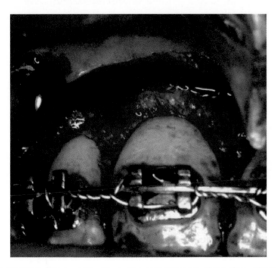

Fig. 2.154 Flap reflection demonstrates that the alveolar crests are at the cementoenamel junctions of the teeth. Osseous resective therapy is required to attain the desired post-therapeutic soft-tissue levels.

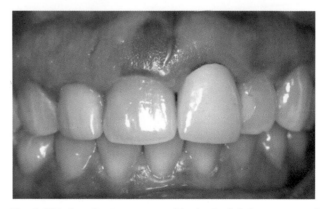

Fig. 2.156 A patient presents with gingival disharmony and incomplete passive eruption. Adequate keratinized tissues are present to enable subsulcular incisions at the desired final soft-tissue positions without jeopardizing the amount of postsurgical keratinized gingiva.

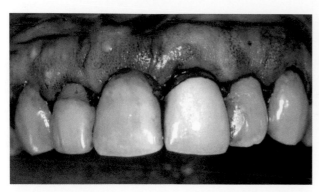

Fig. 2.157 Subsulcular incisions are made to the desired final soft-tissue levels.

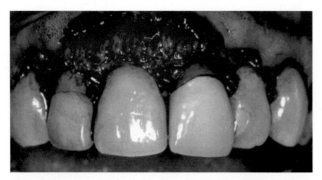

Fig. 2.158 Flap reflection demonstrates that the alveolar crest is within 2 mm of the cementoenamel junctions of the teeth, and that significant buccal alveolar ledging is present.

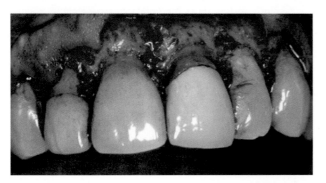

Fig. 2.159 Osseous resective therapy is carried out to eliminate buccal ledging, attain the desired dimension of 2.5 mm from alveolar crest to cementoenamel junctions, and ensure positive osseous architecture.

out to eliminate buccal ledging, establish the necessary 3 mm of dimension between the cementoenamel junctions of the teeth and the alveolar crest, and attain positive osseous architecture (Fig. 2.159). Following healing, gingival harmony is

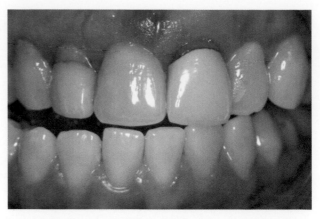

Fig. 2.160 Following healing, gingival harmony has been attained, and no probing depths are present in excess of 2 mm.

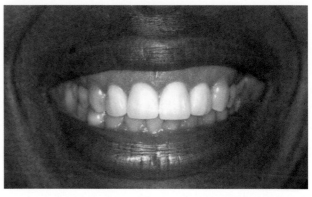

Fig. 2.161 Twenty-six years post-therapy the attained soft-tissue positions and gingival health have been maintained.

attained and all soft-tissue pocketing is eliminated. No probing depths are present in excess of 2 mm (Fig. 2.160). Twenty-six years post-therapy, the patient demonstrates continuing gingival health, and maintenance of the surgically attained soft-tissue positions (Fig. 2.161).

CLINICAL EXAMPLE SIXTEEN

A patient presents with incomplete passive eruption and subgingival decay around restorative dentistry, which had been placed in the maxillary anterior region (Fig. 2.162). Flap reflection reveals the extent of the recurrent caries, and the need to establish biologic width between the caries and the osseous crest on the mesial aspects of teeth numbers 8 and 9 (Fig. 2.163). Following osseous resective therapy, the buccal mucoperiosteal flap is

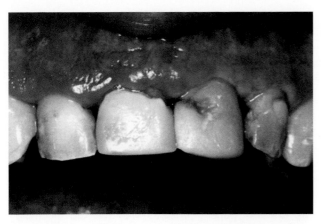

Fig. 2.162 A patient presents with incomplete passive eruption and subgingival caries in the maxillary anterior region.

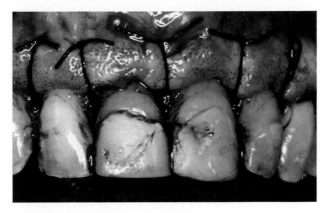

Fig. 2.164 Following appropriate osseous resective therapy, the buccal mucoperiosteal flap is sutured at the desired level.

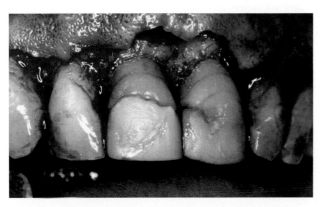

Fig. 2.163 Flap reflection demonstrates the need to establish biologic width between the caries and the alveolar crest on the mesial aspects of the maxillary central incisors. Note that the palatal soft tissues have been maintained.

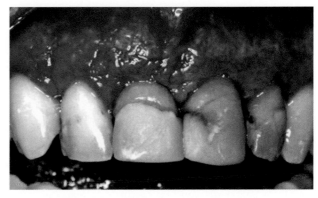

Fig. 2.165 Post-therapeutically, the desired soft-tissue levels and contours have been attained, the interproximal papillae have been maintained, and all caries is supragingival and accessible for appropriate restorative intervention.

sutured at osseous crest (Fig. 2.164). As the caries does not extend to the palatal aspects of the teeth and there is no incomplete passive eruption palatally, a palatal flap was not reflected and the palatal aspects of the interproximal soft tissues were maintained, in an attempt to avoid development of "black holes" between the teeth post-therapy. Following appropriate healing, desired soft-tissue contours have been attained, the interproximal papillae are still intact, and all caries and older restorative therapy are supragingival and accessible for appropriate intervention (Fig. 2.165).

When working in the aesthetic zone, should concomitant palatal IPE be noted, submarginal crestally anticipated incisions are employed, flaps are

reflected, and osseous therapy is performed as necessary to provide 2.5 mm from the osseous crests to the cementoenamel junctions of the teeth to be treated. In such a situation, the interproximal soft tissues are not debrided. Once again, they are left in place, attached, to help preserve the interproximal papillae (Figs. 2.166–2.168).

Failure to recognize and treat both the level of the osseous crest with relation to the cementoenamel junction and buccal osseous ledging, so as to both anticipate and participate in final soft-tissue healing, will result in regrowth of soft tissues to a level more coronal than desired, leading to a compromised treatment outcome and patient dissatisfaction. However, when the hard and soft

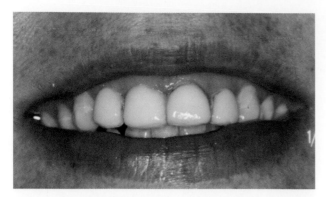

Fig. 2.166 A patient presents with buccal and palatal incomplete passive eruption, and old bonded restorations on the maxillary anterior teeth.

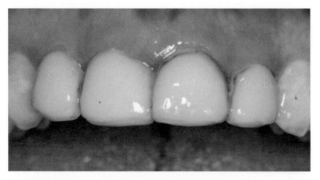

Fig. 2.167 A close-up demonstrates recurrent caries around much of the older restorative dentistry that had been placed, and the marked incomplete passive eruption that is present.

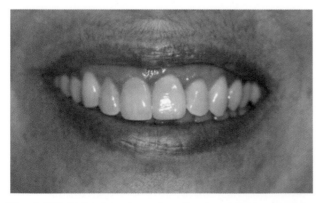

Fig. 2.168 Following crown-lengthening osseous surgery with retention of the interproximal soft tissues, the desired final buccal soft-tissue positions have been attained, and restorative therapy has been carried out. Note the maintenance of the interproximal soft-tissue papillae.

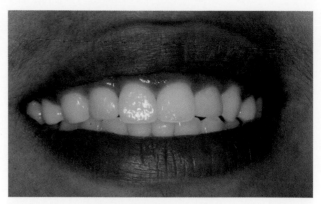

Fig. 2.169 A patient presents with marked incomplete passive eruption and aesthetic dissatisfaction. Note the delicate nature of the interproximal soft tissues. Care must be taken not to disrupt these tissues, so as to avoid interproximal tissue recession and an unaesthetic final-treatment result.

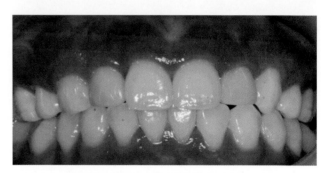

Fig. 2.170 A close-up view demonstrates incomplete passive eruption, thin keratinized tissues, and the delicate interproximal soft tissues that are present.

tissues are managed appropriately, the final treatment result is significant improvement of the aesthetic profile and periodontal health, and a high degree of patient satisfaction (Figs. 2.169–2.171).

INDICATIONS AND CONTRAINDICATIONS FOR CROWN-LENGTHENING SURGERY

It is imperative to recognize the indications and contraindications for crown-lengthening osseous surgery (see Tables 2.1, 2.2; see also discussion in Chapter 6).

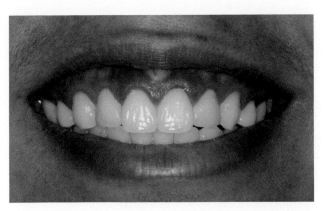

Fig. 2.171 Following crown-lengthening surgery, the desired soft-tissue margins have been attained, and the interproximal soft tissues have been maintained. The result is a high degree of patient satisfaction.

Table 2.1. Indications for crown-lengthening surgery.

Indications
Subgingival caries
Subgingival tooth fracture
Deeply subgingival restorations
Inadequate tooth structure for proper retention
Inadequate tooth height for establishment of proper clinical crown contours
Crown proximity problems due to tooth tilting, which have led to embrasure space concerns
Need to perform odontoplasty to improve tooth emergence and/or eliminate incipient or Class I furcation involvements
Incomplete passive eruption
Aesthetic concerns with "short teeth"
Aesthetic concerns with lack of gingival marginal harmony

Indications

Subgingival Caries

In all instances where the tooth is to be maintained, either the hard and/or soft tissue should be recontoured, or the tooth should be supererupted prior to such recontouring in order to render all

Table 2.2. Contraindications for crown-lengthening surgery.

Contraindications
Systemic factors which preclude surgery
Teeth with significantly reduced osseous support
Teeth with untreatable periodontal osseous defects
Periodontally hopeless teeth
Teeth with untreatable furcation involvements
Nonrestorable teeth
Endodontically untreatable teeth
The need to remove extensive osseous support from adjacent teeth
Teeth with inadequate anatomic root length
Teeth with short root trunks

caries supragingival and accessible both for appropriate restorative intervention and for establishment of a restorative margin that can be predictably maintained by the patient. The decision must be made whether to affect such crown-lengthening surgery through use of externally beveled incisions or lasers, or to employ flap reflection with osseous resection as previously described.

If at least 4 mm of dimension exist between the planned restorative margin and the crest of bone, and osseous ledging is not present in such a position as to dictate that the soft tissues will heal more coronally than desired, either a gingivectomy or laser approach may be employed to effect crown-lengthening osseous surgery (Flow Chart 2.1). However, if less than 4 mm of dimension are present between the planned restorative margin and the bone crest, problematic osseous ledging is present, or a concave interproximal soft-tissue col form has developed due to the soft tissues having to "dip under" the contact points, flap reflection with appropriate osseous recontouring must be carried out, as previously described. If there is a doubt as to the need for crown-lengthening osseous surgery, a flap approach should be utilized. External incisions or lasers should be employed only when the clinician is positive that neither of the aforementioned complicating factors is present.

Subgingival Tooth Fracture

Crown-lengthening osseous surgery is always necessary in the face of subgingival tooth fracture. To assume that such a fracture would occur in a position that leaves 4 mm between the point of planned restorative margin apical to the fracture and the osseous crest, and that the fracture is in a position so as not to require osseous recontouring at any point in its three-dimensional consideration, is ill-advised. Neither the patient nor the clinician is well served by performing an excisional technique, restoring the tooth, and having a treatment outcome that is compromised with regard to patient plaque control from the onset.

Deeply Subgingival Restorations

Even if no caries is evident, and no significant bone and attachment loss have occurred in the presence of deep subgingival restorations, such a situation is not maintainable. It is only a question of when the increased plaque accumulation at the restorative margin tooth interface, in a position that is not accessible to the patient for appropriate home-care efforts, will help initiate both periodontitis, and caries at the restorative margin-tooth interface. It is certainly not logical to perform crown-lengthening osseous surgery on an elderly patient who demonstrates subgingival restorations and no active disease. However, such actuarial concerns aside, a patient who presents with deeply subgingival restorations should be treated appropriately through crown-lengthening periodontal surgery, to establish a healthy periodontal milieu and to help improve the long-term prognoses of the restorations that are in place, and thus the teeth.

Inadequate Tooth Structure for Proper Retention

The literature is replete with suggested techniques to help improve retention of restorations on "short teeth." Proponents of such procedures suggest grooves in the teeth, insertion of pins, and other techniques. Such problems are more simply and predictably treated through the performance of crown-lengthening osseous surgery. In addition, the final treatment outcome will demonstrate a much improved long-term prognosis. Once again, if the planned restorative margin is at least 4 mm from the osseous crest in all dimensions, and if no

osseous ledging is present that would contribute to a more coronal postoperative soft-tissue position than desired or the development of a concave interproximal soft-tissue col form, an incisional/laser approach may be employed. However, such an approach should be chosen with great caution and after an extremely rigorous selection process.

Inadequate Tooth Height for Establishment of Proper Clinical Crown Contours

Clearly, this problem is easily solved through appropriate crown-lengthening osseous surgery, as previously discussed.

Crown Proximity Problems Due to Tooth Tilting, Which Have Led to Embrasure Space Concerns

Rather than attempting to place a restoration in a nonideal embrasure space, which will prove difficult if not impossible for the patient to maintain, crown-lengthening osseous surgery should be employed with odontoplasty, as already outlined. Such odontoplasty will not help to solve root proximity problems, which must be dealt with orthodontically. However, when the problem is one of anatomic crown proximity, odontoplasty in conjunction with crown-lengthening osseous surgery will predictably resolve the clinical quandary.

The Need to Perform Odontoplasty to Improve Tooth Emergence and/or Eliminate Incipient or Class I Furcation Involvements

It is imperative that incipient and Class I furcation involvements be eliminated prior to final restoration. Failure to do so will leave the patient with a cul de sac, which will harbor plaque and continue to break down. Elimination of such furcation involvements is easily accomplished through the use of odontoplasty to the osseous crest, as will be discussed in Chapter 3. In addition, odontoplasty should be utilized to alter emergence profiles on posterior teeth which will receive full coverage restorations. Such alteration, so as to provide a flatter (more perpendicular) emergence profile as the tooth exits the osseous crest, will help control the soft tissue at the tooth bone interface, prevent tissue pileup on a microclinical level, and further aid in plaque control efforts.

Incomplete Passive Eruption

As discussed, incomplete passive eruption is both a health and aesthetic concern. As such, it is important that pseudopocketing be eliminated. The decision regarding whether or not to use an excisional/laser approach or a flap approach with or without osseous recontouring has been previously discussed, and is detailed in Flow Chart 2.1.

Aesthetic Concerns with "Short Teeth"

Once again, appropriate decision making is detailed in Flow Chart 2.1.

Aesthetic Concerns with Lack of Gingival Marginal Harmony

Minor cases of gingival margin inconsistency are easily treated through use of a gingivectomy/laser technique. However, care must be taken to ascertain the position of the alveolar crest and the presence or absence of buccal osseous ledging prior to employing such a technique, so as to avoid patient dissatisfaction and embarrassment with the final treatment outcome. This topic has been discussed in detail when addressing incomplete passive eruption.

Contraindications

Contraindications for crown-lengthening osseous surgery include the following.

Systemic Factors

Patients who are ill suited for surgical intervention should not be treated. However, such considerations are not the focus of our discussion.

Teeth with Significantly Reduced Osseous Support

If crown-lengthening osseous surgery will weaken the tooth to such an extent as to cause significant mobility, induce secondary occlusal trauma, or otherwise compromise the tooth's long-term prognosis, crown-lengthening osseous surgery should not be contemplated. In such a situation, tooth extraction and replacement with an implant and crown are often the most appropriate treatments of choice, as will be discussed in Chapter 6.

Teeth with Untreatable Periodontal Osseous Defects

If the osseous defects that are present cannot be predictably eliminated either through osseous resective surgical techniques or through a combination of osseous resection to reduce the defects and regenerative therapy, the tooth is ill suited for crown-lengthening osseous surgery and subsequent restoration. Once again, such a tooth is best treated through removal and replacement.

Periodontally Hopeless Teeth

Teeth that have been deemed to have a poor periodontal prognosis are not candidates for surgical intervention and subsequent restoration, in light of the more predictable regenerative and implant therapeutic modalities that are now available.

Teeth with Untreatable Furcation Involvements

A furcation involvement is deemed treatable if both its horizontal and vertical components may be predictably eliminated through resective and/or regenerative therapies, as will be discussed in Chapter 3. If this is not the case, the tooth is a poor candidate for periodontal and restorative therapies.

Nonrestorable Teeth

If restoration of the tooth following crown-lengthening osseous surgery would be problematic, or if such restoration must be carried out in a nonideal manner, the tooth is a poor candidate for retention.

Endodontically Untreatable Teeth

Should there be any questions regarding the ability to successfully endodontically treat a tooth following crown-lengthening osseous surgery, these questions must be resolved prior to embarking upon therapy. If the endodontic prognosis of the tooth is not excellent, the tooth should not be maintained. Endodontic prognosis includes not only the ability to obtain an adequate seal of the apex or apices of the tooth root(s), but also the ability to leave adequate residual tooth structure following access hole preparation and endodontic therapy to allow successful restoration of the tooth without an undue risk of tooth fracture.

The Need to Remove Extensive Osseous Support from Adjacent Teeth

If crown-lengthening osseous surgery on a given tooth will result in significant compromise of the support of adjacent teeth, alternative therapies must be pursued. These alternative therapies could include orthodontic supereruption of the tooth and subsequent crown-lengthening surgery, or tooth removal and replacement with an implant supported crown.

Teeth with Inadequate Anatomic Root Length

If crown-lengthening osseous surgery will result in a poor crown/root ratio, which will compromise the long-term prognosis of the tooth and/or induce secondary occlusal trauma, the tooth is a poor candidate for crown-lengthening osseous surgery.

Teeth with Short Root Trunks

In such a situation, osseous resective therapy to afford appropriate crown length and eliminate osseous defects and establish a positive osseous architecture would result in the creation of furcation involvements on the tooth being treated. When faced with the choices of either maintaining such a tooth in its current state, performing crown-lengthening osseous surgery that creates furcation involvements and restoring the tooth, or removing the tooth and replacing it, the choice is clear. Maintenance of the tooth in its existing state is not an option, as obvious problems are present that required crown-lengthening osseous surgery. Creating furcation involvements and then restoring the now compromised tooth is a poor option. Tooth removal and replacement with an implant supported crown is the treatment of choice. Which option is chosen will depend upon the clinician's understanding of treatment potentials, and individual clinical acumen.

Conclusion

Failure to comprehensively deal with the periodontal and restorative aspects of the embrasure space will result in a poor long-term prognosis and a higher incidence of periodontal and restorative complications. However, through proper consideration and treatment of the osseous, gingival, and tooth components of the embrasure space, the clinician is able to deliver to the patient a predictable, more easily maintained environment for the reception of restorative dentistry (Flow Chart 2.2).

References

1. Leon AR. The periodontium and restorative procedures. A critical review. J Oral Rehabil 1977;4:105–17.
2. Waerhaug J. Histologic considerations which govern where the margins of restorations should be located in relation to the gingiva. Dent Clin North Am 1960; 161–67.
3. Bjorn AL, et al. Marginal fit of restorations and its relation to periodontal bone level. I. Metal fillings. Odontologisk Revy 1969;20:311.
4. Renggli H, Regolati B. Gingival inflammation and plaque accumulation by well-adapted subgingival and supragingival proximal restorations. Helv Odontol Acta 1972;159:99–101.
5. Leon AR. Amalgam restorations and periodontal disease. Brit Dent J 1976;140:377–82.
6. Jeffcoat MK, Howell TH. Alveolar bone destruction due to overhanging amalgam in periodontal disease. J Periodontol 1980;51:599–602.
7. Keszthely G, Szabo I. Influence of class II amalgam filling on attachment loss. J Clin Periodontol 1984;11: 81–86.
8. Gorzo I, et al. Amalgam restorations. I. Plaque removal and periodontal health. J Clin Periodontol 1979;6: 98–105.
9. Rodriguez-Ferrer H, et al. Effect on gingival health of removing overhanging margins of interproximal subgingival amalgam restorations. J Clin Periodontol 1980;7:457–62.
10. Fugazzotto PA. Comprehensive surgical management of the embrasure space in the prosthetic patient. J Mass Dent Soc 1998;46:18–22.
11. Löe H, Silness J. Tissue reactions to the string packs used in fixed restorations. J Prosthet Dent 1963;13: 318–34.
12. Duncan JD. Reaction of marginal gingiva to crown and bridge procedures. Part 1. J Miss Dent Assoc 1979;35: 26–28.
13. Dragoo MR, Williams GB. Periodontol tissue reactions to restorative procedures. Int J. Periodontics Restorative Dent 1981;1:8–23.
14. Fugazzotto PA, Parma-Benfenati S. Preprosthetic periodontal considerations. Crown length and biologic width. Quint Internat 1984;15:1247–56.

15. Parma-Benfenati S, Fugazzotto PA, Ruben MP. The effect of restorative margins on the post-surgical development and nature of the periodontium. Int J Periodontics Restorative Dent 1985;5: 31–51.
16. Ruben MP, et al. Healing of periodontal surgical wounds. In: Goldman HM, Cohen WD, editors. Periodontal therapy. 6th ed. St. Louis: C.V. Mosby Co., 1980.
17. Carnevale G, Sterrantino SF, DiFebo G. Soft- and hard-tissue wound healing following tooth preparation to the alveolar crest. Int J Periodontics Restorative Dent 1983;3:37–53.
18. Bukrinsky S. A histologic study of the role of periosteum in the attachment of free autogenous gingival grafts to cortical bone. Int J Periodontics Restorative Dent 1985;5:60–63.
19. Pfeifer J. The growth of gingival tissues over bone. J Periodontol 1965;36:36–39.
20. Friedman N. Mucogingival surgery: The apically positioned flap. J Periodontol 1962;33:328–34.

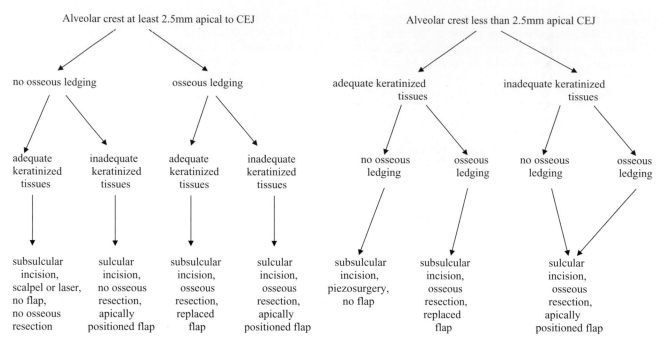

Flow chart 2.1 Treating incomplete passive eruption.

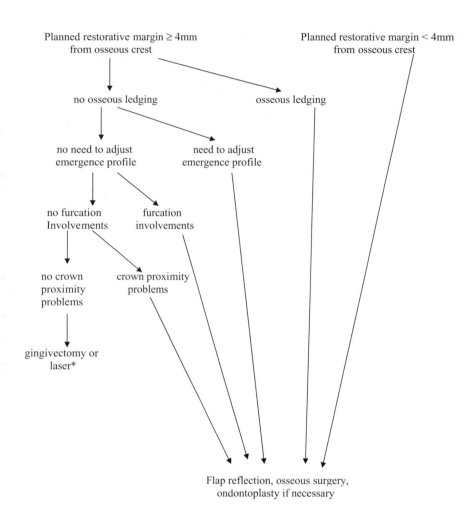

*clinical scenario occurs 1-2% of the time

Flow chart 2.2 Choosing a treatment approach for crown-lengthening surgery.

Chapter 3
Treating the Periodontally Involved Furcation

Paul Fugazzotto

Assuming that all other pocketing around a given molar may be eliminated and necessary crown length gained through appropriate periodontal osseous resective surgery, should buccal and/or lingual furcation involvements of the tooth be treated? Is it necessary to eliminate such furcation involvements? These questions must be answered before determining the fate of, or carrying out restorative therapy on, any periodontally involved bicuspid or molar.

Definitions of Furcation Involvements

When faced with a periodontally involved furcation, treatment decisions must be made in the context of an appropriate definition of therapeutic success. As already discussed, successful periodontal therapy is not characterized by short-term clinical health and immediate gratification. The net result of successful periodontal therapy should be an ease of patient maintenance, long-term predictability, and tooth retention in a healthy state for as long as possible. Predictability is defined as stable attachment levels and no continued loss of supporting bone or periodontal attachment.

Specific patient considerations may impact this definition of success. When considering a patient of advanced age, or one whose medical status is a contraindication to performing the desired therapy, compromises in the above definitions of success must be accepted. However, this discussion will assume no medical contraindications to therapy, and will ignore actuarial considerations.

The challenges confronting the concerned clinician when considering periodontal health, whether he or she is a periodontist or a restorative dentist, are well documented. Deeper pocket depths are less conducive to plaque control efforts and the maintenance of oral health than shallower pocket depths. The literature has reported that deeper pocket depths should be viewed as having greater potential for future periodontal breakdown than shallower pocket depths. Furcation involvements have been shown to represent a unique and challenging area of potential plaque accumulation and rapid periodontal breakdown. Numerous authors have demonstrated that the presence of furcation involvements may be utilized as a predictor for future attachment loss around the tooth in question.

The definitions of success following furcation therapy must be stringent and clinically relevant. Failure to wholly eliminate the horizontal and vertical components of a furcation involvement and thus the inability to provide the patient with a milieu that is conducive to maximum effectiveness of home-care efforts, must be deemed unsatisfactory. The appropriate definition of success following furcation therapy is elimination of all horizontal and vertical components of the furcation involvement, and no probing depths in excess of 3 mm on any aspects of the tooth in question.

The treatment approach chosen, whether it be resection, regeneration, a combination of resection and regeneration, or tooth removal and implant placement, is dependent upon the involved furcation morphology. It is therefore critical that easy-to-use, clinically applicable definitions of furcation involvements be employed to aid in the development of appropriate treatment algorithms.

Furcation defects are described as a function of the extent of periodontal destruction in both the

Periodontal Restorative Interrelationships: Ensuring Clinical Success, First Edition. Edited by Paul A. Fugazzotto.
© 2011 by John Wiley & Sons, Inc. Published 2011 by John Wiley & Sons, Inc.

horizontal and vertical dimensions. Horizontal furcation involvements are defined as follows:

A. Class I: Entrance into the furcation proceeds less than half of the horizontal dimension of the tooth (Fig. 3.1).
B. Class II: Entrance into the furcation proceeds greater that half of the horizontal dimension of the tooth, but less than the full horizontal dimension of the tooth (Fig. 3.2).
C. Class III: Entrance into the furcation proceeds along the complete horizontal dimension of the tooth, connecting both the buccal and lingual furcation entrances (Fig. 3.3).

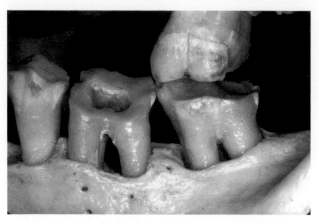

Fig. 3.3 Class III furcation involvements are noted on both the first and second molars.

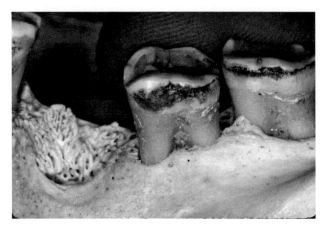

Fig. 3.1 Class I furcation involvements are noted on both molars.

Vertical furcation involvements are defined as follows:

A. Subclass a: Loss of attachment apparatus along less than 25% of the vertical component of the furcation of the tooth.
B. Subclass b: Loss of attachment apparatus along more than 25% but less than 50% of the vertical component of the furcation of the tooth.
C. Subclass c: Loss of attachment apparatus along more than 50% of the vertical component of the furcation of the tooth.

Although the vertical component of a furcation involvement has significant ramifications in the treatment of Class II furcations, it plays a minimal role in the treatment of Class I furcations, unless the vertical involvement either extends to such a degree as to render attainment of appropriate osseous morphologies impossible, or reaches the apices of the tooth in question. In such situations, regenerative therapy or molar extraction and implant placement must be effected, depending upon the extent of the problem.

Examination of the root morphologies facing involved periodontal furcations demonstrates the difficulty, and often futility, of attempting to thoroughly debride these areas through the use of curettes and/or ultrasonic instrumentation, either through a closed or open-flap approach (Fig. 3.4). Molars presenting with additional roots, whether they be fully formed or vestigial in nature, pose an even greater challenge to the treating clinician (Fig. 3.5).

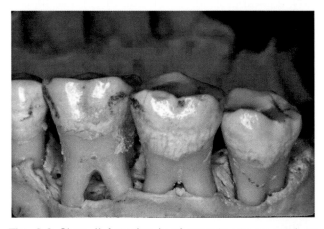

Fig. 3.2 Class II furcation involvements are present on both the first and second molars. The greater vertical component of the furcation involvement on the first molar renders treatment of this area more problematic than the Class II furcation on the second molar.

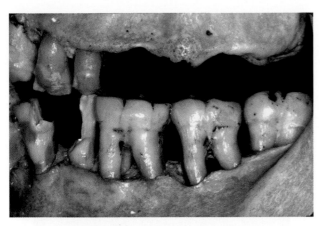

Fig. 3.4 The morphologies of the root surfaces facing a periodontally involved furcation on a mandibular molar render appropriate debridement difficult, if not impossible.

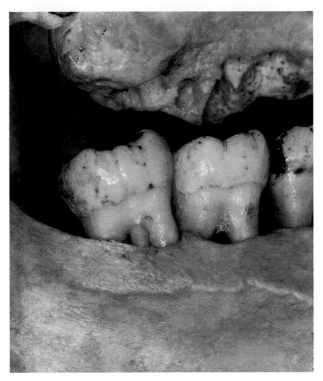

Fig. 3.5 The presence of an additional root complicates debridement of the periodontally involved furcation of the second molar.

A comprehensive review of the literature conclusively demonstrates that reduction of post-therapeutic pocket depths and the establishment of a stable, predictable attachment apparatus will result in a greater degree of long-term periodontal success with regard to the maintenance of oral health and the prevention of repocketing and reinitiation of periodontal disease processes.

An appropriate review of the literature also underscores the inadequacy of many therapies in the predictable treatment of the furcated tooth. "Maintenance" care, open-flap and closed-flap debridement of the furcation, chemical treatment of the root surfaces facing the involved furcation, and placement of various particulate materials without covering membranes or growth factors have failed to demonstrate predictable success in the treatment of the periodontally involved furcation.

Use of covering nonresorbable and resorbable membranes to treat involved furcations has traditionally met with a varying degree of success, although strict diagnostic criteria and a number of technical modifications to the conventional techniques will yield a high degree of success in the treatment of Class II buccal furcation involvements. The use of platelet derived growth factors and a number of other growth factors shows great promise in effecting regeneration of damaged bone and attachment apparatus in the periodontal involved furcation. However, this is not the forum in which to discuss such therapies.

It is critical to realize that certain therapeutic approaches are inadequate in the treatment of furcations of varying degrees of involvement, while other approaches are predictable and straightforward in resolving the problems associated with early furcation involvements.

There is no doubt that periodontally involved furcations may not be predictably maintained through root planing and curettage and repeated maintenance care sessions. In a longitudinal study of patients who refused active periodontal therapy and underwent only continuing maintenance care, Becker et al. (1) reported an overall rate of tooth loss of 9.8% in the mandible and 11.4% in the maxilla. Patients demonstrated a rate of tooth loss of 22.5% for mandibular furcated teeth and 17% for maxillary teeth with furcation involvements. These findings underscore the fact that teeth with furcation involvements are less amenable to maintenance care than their single-rooted counterparts.

The fact that teeth with furcation involvements are less amenable to maintenance care than their single-rooted counterparts is confirmed by Goldman et al. (2), who assessed tooth loss in 211 patients treated in a private periodontal practice through root planing, curettage, and open-flap debridement, and maintained for 15 to 30 years on a consistent recall schedule. Furcation involvements were not eliminated. The overall rate of tooth loss was 13.4%. Maxillary and mandibular teeth with furcation involvements were lost at a rate of 30.7% and 24.2%, respectively, a rate that was significantly higher than the incidence of non-furcated tooth loss.

McFall (3) reported on tooth loss in 100 treated patients with periodontal disease, who were maintained for 15 years or longer following active periodontal therapy. Once again, therapy did not eliminate the furcation involvements that were present. Of all teeth, 11.3% were lost over the course of observation. Maxillary teeth that demonstrated furcation involvements were lost at a rate of 22.3% over the course of this study. Mandibular furcated teeth were lost at a rate of 14.7%. Similar finding are reported throughout the literature (4–6).

As with other therapies, appropriate treatment of involved furcations depends upon many factors that are common to all aspects of dentistry. These include proper patient selection, establishment of adequate plaque control, formulation of a comprehensive overall treatment plan, and other factors previously discussed. However, a periodontally involved furcation also presents unique challenges that demand innovative treatment approaches and a realistic assessment of when to maintain a furcated tooth and when the tooth must be removed and replaced.

A study by Fleisher et al. (7) underscores the fallacy of believing that complete debridement of a periodontally involved furcation may be accomplished utilizing curettes and ultrasonic instrumentation. Fifty molars were treated through either closed curettage or open-flap debridement. All teeth were treated by experienced operators. The teeth were then extracted and stained for the presence of plaque and/or calculus. Assessment of the extracted and stained teeth demonstrated that only 68% of the tooth surfaces facing the involved furcation were calculus free.

While there is no doubt that the utilization of microscopy and appropriate instrumentation will greatly improve upon this level of efficacy of furcation debridement, the three-dimensional structure of the involved furcation will remain (Fig. 3.6). The net result will be repopulation of this area by plaque, and reinitiation of a periodontal inflammatory lesion. Such an approach will "slow down"

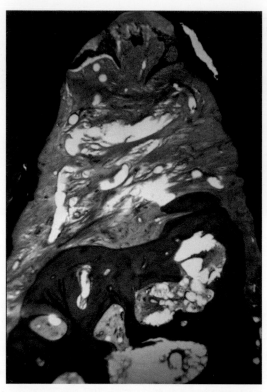

Fig. 3.6 Debridement of a furcation area, without elimination of the physical aspects of the furcation involvement bordered by the roots and the alveolar bone, does not halt the active disease process.

the progression of bone and attachment loss, and may prove valuable in an older patient or one who cannot or will not undergo more comprehensive therapy. However, such a treatment endpoint is not desirable in most other clinical scenarios. Therapy must be aimed at eliminating the periodontally involved furcation and providing the patient with a milieu that is amenable to appropriate plaque control efforts and reception of restorative therapy.

Cementoenamel projections represent another potential compromise in both periodontal health and periodontal treatment outcomes. Cementoenamel projections prevent the establishment of a connective-tissue attachment to the root surface, as connective-tissue attachment to enamel is not possible. As a result, these enamel projections are a potential funnel for bacteria into the entrance of the furcation, as the only barrier to such bacterial penetration is an overlying junctional epithelial adhesion.

As discussed in Chapter 1, epithelial adhesion has been shown to unzip in the face of a plaque front and the resultant inflammatory insult. A Class I cementoenamel projection, which extends less than 25% of the root trunk toward the furcation entrance, poses little concern with regard to periodontal health (Fig. 3.7). However, a Class II cementoenamel projection, which extends more than 50% of the dimension of the root trunk toward the furcation entrance but does not actually reach the furcation entrance, should be viewed as a weak link to the fiber-attachment periodontal defense system (Fig. 3.8). A Class III cementoenamel projection, which by definition extends to or into the entrance of the furcation, is an absolute compromise to periodontal health, as no connective-tissue attachment is present between the gingival sulcus and the entrance to the furcation (Fig. 3.9). Patients with such an abnormality are literally born with

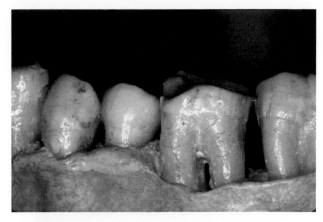

Fig. 3.9 A Class III cementoenamel projection is present on the first molar.

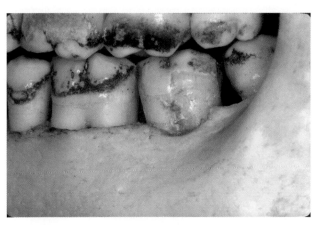

Fig. 3.7 A Class I cementoenamel projection is present on the first molar.

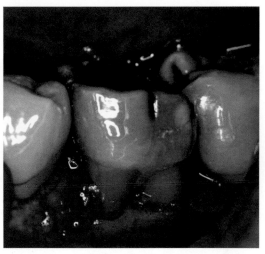

Fig. 3.10 Flap reflection reveals a Class III cementoenamel projection with the expected furcation involvement. The inability of the body to develop a connective tissue attachment to enamel renders this tooth highly susceptible to continued periodontal breakdown in the furcation area.

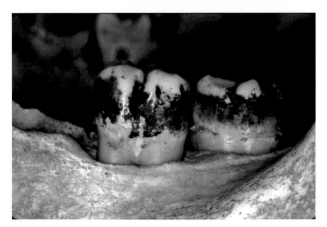

Fig. 3.8 A Class II cementoenamel projection is present on the first molar.

furcation involvements (Fig. 3.10). Failure to treat these areas in a timely and effective manner often leads to significant progression of periodontal disease problems in the furcation area and premature loss of the molar in question. Fig. 3.11 demonstrates a patient who presented with a Class III cementoenamel projection and was not treated through appropriate resective therapy. The result was continued periodontal breakdown. A Class III furcation involvement is now present on the tooth in question, which has a hopeless prognosis. Appropriate, timely intervention would have helped

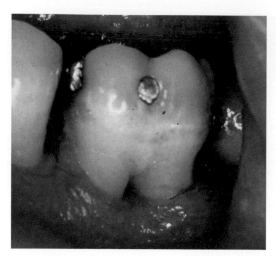

Fig. 3.11 Failure to treat a Class III cementoenamel projection in a timely and effective manner has resulted in the development of Class III furcation involvement and a hopeless prognosis for a mandibular first molar.

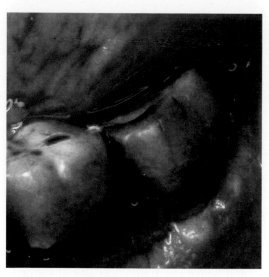

Fig. 3.13 The enamel pearl in the furcation area of the second molar both prohibits development of connective-tissue attachment in the region and serves as a nidus for plaque and calculus accumulation.

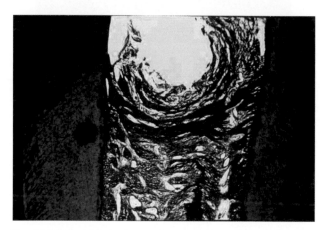

Fig. 3.12 A histologic section of the extracted tooth demonstrates both connective-tissue attachment to the cementum-covered root surfaces facing the furcation, and the lack of true attachment in the area of the cementoenamel projection.

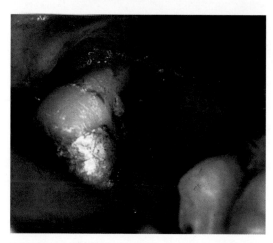

Fig. 3.14 Flap reflection reveals a large enamel pearl at the entrance of the mesial furcation of a maxillary molar. Note the periodontal destruction that has occurred in the area due to the inability to effect appropriate home-care measures.

avoid such a development. The histologic specimen of the extracted tooth demonstrates attachment apparatus on the root surfaces, which were covered with cementum, and a lack of any attachment in the area of the cementoenamel projection (Fig. 3.12).

Enamel pearls are also a significant concern (Figs. 3.13, 3.14). They represent both an area devoid of connective-tissue attachment to the root surface and a morphology that is conducive to plaque accumulation.

Diagnosing Premolar Furcation Involvements

Mesial and distal furcation involvements on maxillary premolars are the most often ignored or misdiagnosed of all furcation entities. In addition, these furcation involvements pose unique dangers to overall periodontal health. An ignored mesial

Class I furcation involvement on a maxillary first premolar, if allowed to progress, will result in significant loss of alveolar bone and attachment apparatus not only around the tooth in question, but also on the distal aspect of the adjacent cuspid (Figs. 3.15– 3.17). Such a development may compromise the integrity of the quadrant, or condemn a previously fabricated long-span fixed prosthesis. It is imperative that the furcation entrances of maxillary premolars be examined, diagnosed, and managed properly, to ensure long-term periodontal and restorative health.

Treatment of Class I Furcations

The horizontal components of Class I furcation involvements may always be eliminated through ondontoplasty. If bone loss in the area of the Class I furcation involvement has a vertical component, which extends to such an extent that positive osseous architecture may not be developed, the problems in this region cannot be resolved through odontoplasty. Fortunately, such developments are rare with Class I furcation involvements. The roof of the furcation is recontoured to eliminate the cul de sac, which traps plaque, and the newly established tooth contours are carried onto the radicular surfaces of the tooth to create a continuous, smooth morphology conducive to patient plaque control efforts. Pocket-elimination surgery

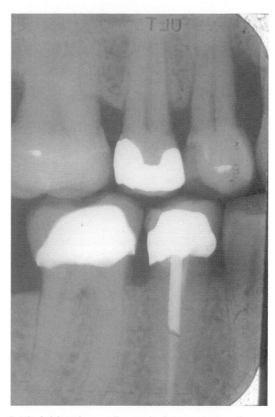

Fig. 3.16 A bitewing radiograph demonstrates the severe loss of bone and attachment apparatus which has taken place on the mesial aspect of the maxillary first bicuspid.

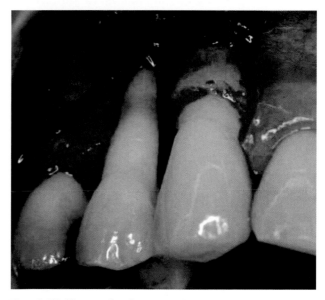

Fig. 3.17 Flap reflection reveals severe osseous loss around the maxillary first bicuspid. This tooth is now hopeless. Timely intervention when the furcation involvement first began to develop would have avoided this problem.

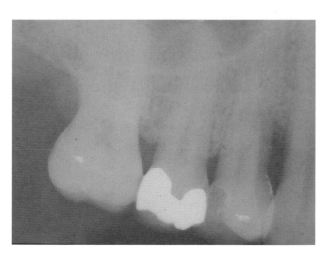

Fig. 3.15 A patient presents with a 7-mm pocket on the mesial aspect of the maxillary first bicuspid. The patient has been under regular maintenance care at another office.

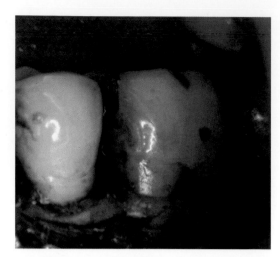

Fig. 3.18 The patient presents with a Class I buccal furcation involvement and a Class II cementoenamel projection.

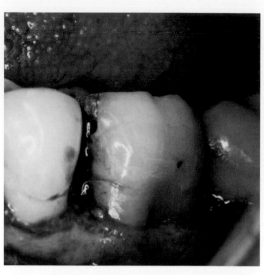

Fig. 3.19 Following appropriate odontoplasty, the cementoenamel projection has been removed and the Class I furcation involvement has been eliminated. Mucoperiosteal flaps will now be sutured at osseous crest. The net result of treatment will be an area that is easily maintained by the patient.

employing osseous resection with apically positioned flaps is performed at the same time. The net results of treatment are the elimination of deeper pocket depths and Class I furcation involvements. The post-therapeutic definition of success is no entrance of the probe into the furcation of the tooth and no probing depths in excess of 3 mm around the tooth. Coincident to the performed ondontoplasty is the elimination of all cementoenamel projections, thus enhancing the ability to form an appropriate attachment apparatus to protect the furcal entrance (Figs. 3.18, 3.19).

CLINICAL EXAMPLE ONE

A patient presents having been temporized throughout the maxillary arch in anticipation of placing individual full-coverage restorations. Significant pocket depths had been noted on the mesial aspect of the maxillary first bicuspid. Flap reflection demonstrates a Class I furcation involvement (Fig. 3.20). The following treatment options must be considered by the clinician:

- *"Maintenance" of the Class I furcation involvement through repeated scaling and root planing*: As already discussed, this treatment approach will not halt the disease process. The net result will be continued bone and attachment loss in the area, jeopardizing both the first bicuspid and the cuspid.
- *Extraction of the first bicuspid and placement of a three-unit fixed splint, extending from the*

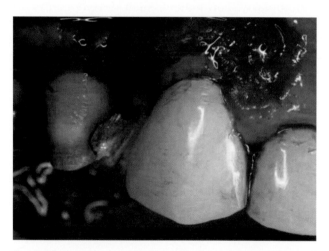

Fig. 3.20 A patient presents with all maxillary teeth provisionalized for individual full-coverage restorations. Note the Class I furcation involvement on the mesial aspect of the maxillary first bicuspid. Failure to treat this area will severely compromise the long-term prognoses of the first bicuspid and cuspid.

second bicuspid to the cuspid: Such a treatment option poses two concerns. The first is that, if regenerative therapy is not performed at the time of tooth extraction, collapse of the socket and loss of some interproximal bone on the distal aspect of the cuspid and the mesial aspect of the second bicuspid are to be expected. The second concern is the greater difficulty in exhibiting appropriate home-care efforts around a three-unit fixed bridge than around individual crowns.

- *Extraction of the first bicuspid with concomitant bone regeneration therapy and placement of a three-unit fixed splint, extending from the second bicuspid to the cuspid*: Although this option addresses the concerns of bone loss subsequent to healing, assuming bone grafting is performed correctly, the concern with regard to increased difficulty of home-care efforts still remains.
- *Extraction of the first premolar with immediate implant insertion and subsequent restoration*: This option is highly predictable. However, there is an additional expense entailed in implant placement and restoration. The question becomes whether or not such therapy is required in this situation.
- *Performance of odontoplasty to eliminate the roof of the involved furcation (Fig. 3.21) and render the area maintainable by the patient*: This option presents with the advantage of

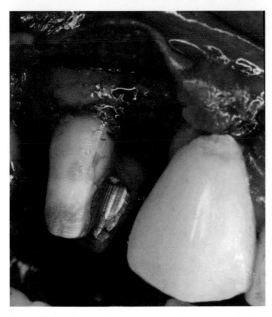

Fig. 3.21 Following odontoplasty, the furcation involvement has been eliminated. Care must now be taken to finish tooth preparation at the gingival margin or slightly intrasulcularly, and to ensure that the contours of the restoration follow the newly created morphology of the tooth at the gingival area.

eliminating the active periodontal problems, as well as the milieu which would help propagate further periodontal disease. In addition, the tooth is maintained, thus lessening the expense to the patient. It is important that the periodontist and restorative dentist communicate regarding the therapy that has been carried out, so that the restorative dentist does not attempt to cover all cut tooth structure, which would result in a restorative margin at the bone crest. In addition, care must be taken to properly contour the final restoration so as not to build in a prosthetic furcation involvement. An in-depth discussion of restorative contours following odontoplasty appears in Chapter 6.

Ondontoplasty is highly predictable and may be carried out without a prosthetic commitment. If all therapy has been performed appropriately to manage osseous contours, including buccal and or palatal/lingual ledging, the attachment apparatus following healing of such therapy consists of approximately 1 mm of connective tissue attachment coronal to the alveolar crest, followed by approximately 1 mm of junctional epithelial adhesion. A 1–2-mm gingival sulcus will be present, against cut tooth structure. Such a minimal probing depth is easily maintainable by the patient, and does not pose a tooth sensitivity problem. After having performed ondontoplasty to eliminate Class I furcation involvements over 20,000 times in 29 years of private practice, only one instance has been encountered where tooth sensitivity persisted beyond 2 weeks post-therapy, unless caries or pulpal pathology had been present prior to treatment. Failure to eradicate early furcation involvements through odontoplasty will result in continued periodontal breakdown and attachment loss in the furcation area, and eventual tooth loss.

Elimination of Class I furcation involvements is conservative therapy. For example, if a 25-year-old patient presents with excellent home care, minimal probing depths, and a Class III cementoenamel projection in the buccal furcation area of a lower first molar, as evidenced by examination following retraction of unattached soft tissues in this area, two treatment approaches may theoretically be considered:

1. The patient could be placed on a strict maintenance schedule, and the clinician could

attempt to maintain the furcation in question through repeated professional prophylaxis visits. The net results of such a treatment approach will be progression of periodontal disease in the furcation area, periodontal attachment loss, and/or development of a deeper furcation involvement.

2. A flap may be reflected, and ondontoplasty performed to eliminate the cementoenamel projection and any early furcation involvements that have developed. The results of such treatment will be elimination of the anatomical factors contributing to periodontal breakdown in the furcation area, the development of an appropriate attachment apparatus, and establishment of hard- and soft-tissue morphologies that are conducive to patient home-care efforts.

Treatment of Class II Furcations

Timely intervention utilizing odontoplasty is crucial when faced with Class I furcation involvements and/or Class III cementoenamel projections, both to preserve the alveolar bone and attachment apparatus around the tooth and to eliminate the need for more aggressive therapies at a later date.

Class II furcation involvements cannot be eliminated through the use of odontoplasty. The resultant tooth contours, characterized by a deep notch in the treated furcation area, would harbor plaque and not be conducive to effective home-care measures (Figs. 3.22, 3.23). When faced with Class II furcation involvements, if the tooth is to be maintained, either resective techniques involving root resection or tooth sectioning, or regenerative techniques employing membranes, graft materials, growth factors or other substances, must be employed. There is no doubt that root-resective and tooth-sectioning techniques are highly effective if performed correctly in the appropriate cases. Such a therapeutic approach is diagnosis and technique sensitive, and mandates a significant financial commitment. The question is whether such a commitment is warranted when we are now able to predictably utilize osseointegrated implants to replace compromised molars.

ROOT RESECTION

While the advent of periodontal regenerative techniques and dental implants has in large part sup-

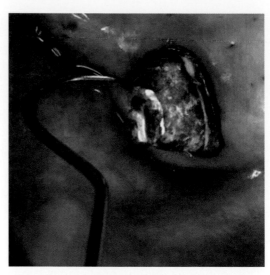

Fig. 3.22 A Class II distal furcation involvement is noted on a maxillary molar.

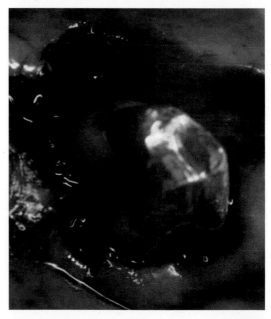

Fig. 3.23 Flap reflection demonstrates attempts to eliminate the furcation involvements on the tooth utilizing odontoplasty. The Class I furcation involvement was easily eliminated through odontoplasty. However, efforts to eliminate the Class II furcation involvement with odontoplasty resulted in a tooth morphology that was not conducive to home-care efforts.

planted the use of root-resective treatment in periodontics, root resection remains a viable treatment alternative, especially in the maxillary molar areas.

CLINICAL EXAMPLE TWO

A patient presents with deep probing on the distal aspect of a maxillary first molar (Fig. 3.24). Flap reflection demonstrates a significant osseous defect, and a Class II distal furcation involvement on the maxillary first molar (Fig. 3.25). Available treatment options include the following:

- *Attempts at maintaining the furcation through repeated scaling and root-planning efforts:*

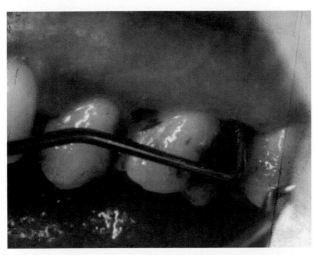

Fig. 3.24 A patient presents with a deep pocket depth on the distobuccal aspect of the maxillary first molar.

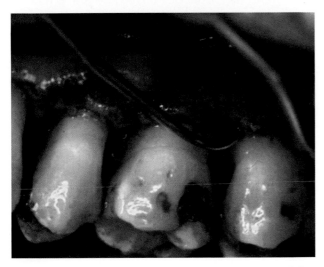

Fig. 3.25 Flap reflection reveals a severe osseous defect between the maxillary first and second molars, and a Class II distal furcation involvement on the maxillary first molar. Any efforts at debridement of this furcation involvement and regenerative therapy would meet with failure.

Such an approach would be ineffective and would lead to continued breakdown of alveolar bone and attachment apparatus in the furcation area and between the two molars, significantly compromising the prognoses of both teeth.

- *Regenerative therapy aimed at rebuilding damaged alveolar bone and attachment apparatus in the aforementioned furcation involvement and infrabony defect areas:* Due to the inability to appropriately debride the Class II distal furcation of the first molar with the second molar in place, regenerative therapy would be ineffective, leading to continued periodontal breakdown in the region.
- *Distobuccal root resection, followed by endodontic therapy and restoration of the first molar (Fig. 3.26):* Such an approach is highly predictable, as has been demonstrated in the literature, assuming other factors are favorable.
- *Extraction of the first molar and regenerative therapy in the socket area. A secondary sinus augmentation procedure may or may not be necessary prior to implant placement and subsequent restoration:* This treatment approach presents with two major disadvantages. The patient is subjected to a number of surgical visits. In addition, the cost of such therapy will be significantly more than attempting to maintain the tooth following root resection, endodontic therapy, and restoration.
- *Extraction of the first molar and placement of an implant with concomitant regenerative*

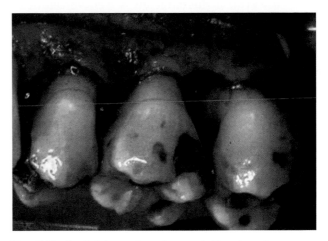

Fig. 3.26 A distobuccal root amputation has been performed on the maxillary first molar.

therapy, if possible: This approach has proven highly predictable, assuming that various criteria are met.

- *Extraction of the maxillary first molar and placement of a three-unit fixed splint*: Such a treatment option poses two concerns. The first is, if no regenerative therapy is done at the time of tooth extraction, collapse of the socket and loss of interproximal bone on the distal aspect of the second bicuspid and the mesial aspect of the second molar are to be expected. The second concern is the greater difficulty in exhibiting appropriate home-care efforts around a three-unit fixed bridge than around individual crowns.
- *Extraction of the maxillary first molar with concomitant regenerative therapy, followed by fabrication of a three-unit fixed splint*: While this option addresses the concerns of bone loss subsequent to healing, assuming bone grafting is carried out correctly, the concern with regard to increased difficulty of home-care efforts still remains.

The therapeutic option chosen will be dependent upon a number of factors including site specific factors, and the comfort of the treating clinician with various modalities. For example, if the clinician is not fluent in the treatment approach which includes tooth extraction, manipulation of the interradicular bone, and placement of an implant with concomitant regenerative therapy in one visit, there will be a greater tendency to look toward either root resection or tooth extraction and fabrication of a three unit fixed splint.

However, if the clinician is well versed in all treatment modalities, a decision can be made which is in the best interest of the patient, regarding whether to resect a root or remove the tooth and place an implant at the time of tooth removal.

Root resection has proven to be a predictable procedure with long lasting results. Multiple clinicians (8–12) have demonstrated long-term success rates with root resection (Table 3.1) that are comparable to other furcation treatments, treatment of single rooted teeth and dental implants.

Nabers et al. (8) treated 1,530 patients with severe periodontal disease and followed them for an average time of 12.9 years post-therapy. All patients were treated with resective periodontal therapy, including furcation elimination through root resection or tooth sectioning. An average of 0.29 teeth were lost over the observation time of the study.

Carnevale et al. (9) assessed the results of resective therapy of 500 sectioned teeth restored and followed for 3–11 years post-treatment. Of these teeth, 94.3% were periodontally healthy and functioning successfully at the end of the observation period.

A paper published in 2001 documented the success and failure of 701 root-resected molars followed for up to 16 years with a mean time in function of 8.1 years (10). The cumulative success rate of the root-resected molars, with success being defined as periodontal stability with no further attachment loss or increase in probing depth, was 96.8%.

However, to attain these levels of predictability, it is imperative that all treating clinicians understand the subtleties of root-resective therapy and its restorative ramifications. As previously mentioned, a thorough diagnosis and comprehensive treatment plan must first be constructed. In addition, various myths and fallacies regarding root-resective therapy must be addressed, critically examined, and dismissed as necessary.

For example, "bicupidization" is a term popularized by proponents of resecting a mandibular molar, retaining both roots, and restoring them as

Table 3.1. Root resection failures over time.

Author(s)	Year published	Observation time	Number of cases treated	Failures (%)
Basten et al. (11)	1996	2–23 years	49	8.0%
Carnevale et al. (10)	1998	10 years	175	7.0%
Fugazzotto (12)	2001	1–16 years	701	3.2%

two bicuspids. Unfortunately, such a course of therapy is usually unrealistic. Figs. 3.27–3.30 demonstrate the impracticality of such a treatment approach. A patient presented with a Class II buccal furcation involvement on a mandibular first molar which had already undergone endodontic therapy (Fig. 3.27). A Class I lingual furcation involvement was also noted (Fig. 3.28). The tooth was hemisected (Fig. 3.29), and the mesial root was extracted (Fig. 3.30). Examination of the interradicular area following removal of the mesial root demonstrated that the sectioning of a mandibular molar does not yield a situation analogous

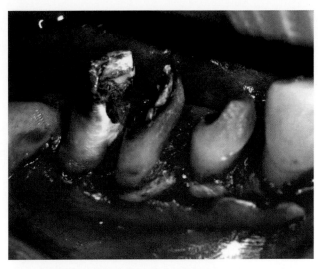

Fig. 3.29 The mandibular first molar has been sectioned. Such "bicuspidization" does not result in two bicuspids.

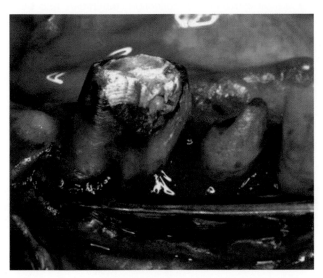

Fig. 3.27 A Class II buccal furcation involvement is present on a mandibular first molar.

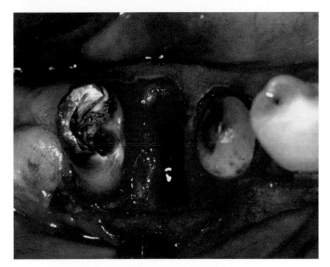

Fig. 3.30 Following extraction of the mesial root of the mandibular first molar, it is evident that a ratio of the buccolingual to mesiodistal dimensions of the interradicular bone between the sectioned roots of the mandibular molar would not have been equal to the same ratio between the two adjacent bicuspids. Retention of both roots of the sectioned mandibular molar would have resulted in a concave col form and an area of difficult maintenance for the patient.

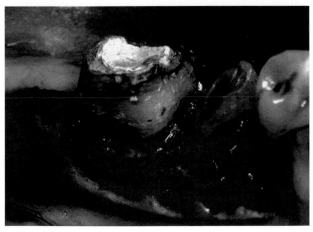

Fig. 3.28 A lingual view demonstrates no periodontal involvement of the lingual furcation of the first molar.

to that of two bicuspids. If a ratio is drawn between the buccolingual dimension of the interproximal space to the mesiodistal dimension of the interproximal space between the two roots of the molar in question, and compared to the same measurements between the adjacent two bicuspids, it becomes obvious that the treatment outcome of bicupidization does not yield an embrasure space as conducive to restoration, appropriate home-care measures, and continued periodontal health as that between two bicuspids. The embrasure space between the two halves of the sectioned molar will demonstrate a concave, nonkeratinized col form, and a greater difficulty in patient home care. The problems inherent in attempting to maintain such a milieu have been discussed in detail in Chapter 2.

If a mandibular molar is to be sectioned, and both roots are to be maintained, orthodontic therapy is usually required to separate the roots, and thus create an embrasure space conducive to long-term periodontal and restorative health.

CLINICAL EXAMPLE THREE

A patient presents with a deep Class II lingual furcation involvement on a mandibular second molar (Fig. 3.31). Following flap reflection, the tooth is sectioned (Fig. 3.32). Subsequent to healing, it is obvious that the embrasure space between the two retained roots will not be conducive to appropriate home-care efforts and maintenance of periodontal health following restoration (Fig. 3.33). The roots are therefore separated orthodontically. Following orthodontic therapy, the embrasure space between the two roots is of such a dimension mesiodistally as to afford the opportunity for appropriate restoration and subsequent home-care efforts (Fig. 3.34).

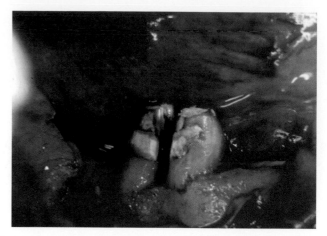

Fig. 3.32 Following flap reflection, the molar has been hemisected.

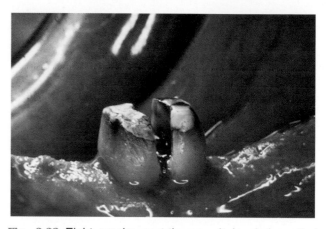

Fig. 3.33 Eight weeks post-therapy, it is obvious that the interproximal area between the two halves of the resected molar is not conducive to appropriate restoration and home-care efforts. The roots will be separated orthodontically.

CLINICAL EXAMPLE FOUR

A patient presents with numerous concerns, including a pulpal floor perforation of the mandibular first molar, a Class II buccal furcation involvement on the mandibular first molar, and inadequate attached keratinized tissue on the buccal aspect of the second bicuspid, an abutment for a planned fixed prosthesis (Fig. 3.35).

Radiographic examination demonstrates moderate root trunk length and good periodontal support around the mandibular first molar (Fig. 3.36). Following flap reflection, the Class II

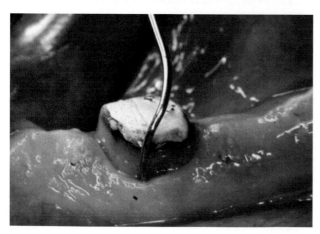

Fig. 3.31 A patient presents with a deep Class II lingual furcation involvement on a mandibular molar.

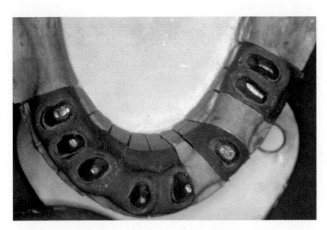

Fig. 3.34 Following orthodontic separation of the hemisected roots, an embrasure space has been created that is ready to receive appropriate restorative therapy, and that is conducive to home-care efforts.

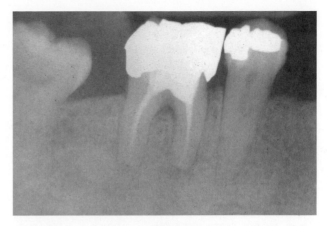

Fig. 3.36 Radiographic examination demonstrates a Class II furcation involvement on the mandibular first molar, and a moderately long root trunk. The periodontal support around the first molar is more than adequate to consider tooth sectioning and root retention.

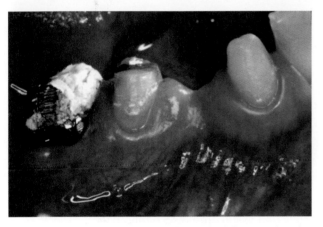

Fig. 3.35 A patient presents with a pulpal floor perforation in the furcation area of the mandibular first molar. In addition, an inadequate band of attached keratinized tissue is evident on the buccal aspect of the second bicuspid.

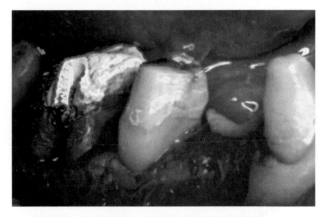

Fig. 3.37 Flap reflection reveals the Class II buccal furcation involvement of the mandibular first molar.

furcation involvement of the first molar is evident (Fig. 3.37). The first molar is hemisected and the mesial root is extracted (Fig. 3.38). Appropriate osseous resective therapy is carried out to ensure the establishment of biologic width around all abutment teeth. Care is also taken to remove any residual tooth "lip" or overhang from the treated furcation area (Fig. 3.39). Prior to flap suturing, a buccal pedicle flap is rotated from the edentulous area between the cuspid and second premolar to the buccal aspect of the second premolar, to help augment the attached keratinized tissue in the region. The flaps are sutured with

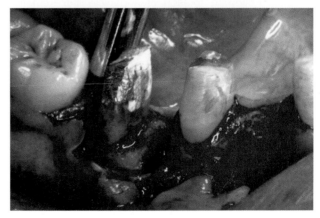

Fig. 3.38 The mandibular first molar has been hemisected and the mesial root extracted.

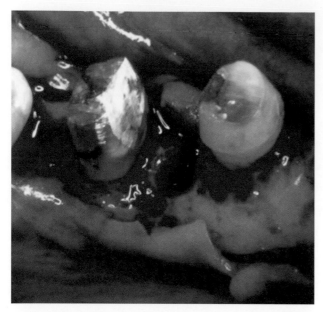

Fig. 3.39 A lingual view demonstrates the elimination of any tooth overhangs in the treated furcation area.

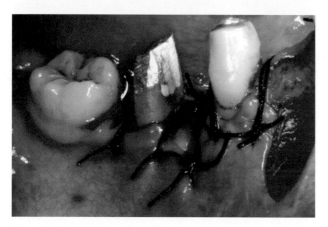

Fig. 3.40 Following rotation of a pedicle flap from the edentulous area to the buccal aspect of the second bicuspid, the mucoperiosteal flaps are sutured with interrupted silk sutures.

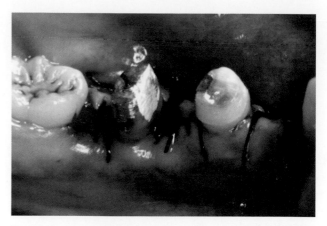

Fig. 3.41 A lingual view demonstrates the crestal anticipation of the lingual flap which had been carried out prior to suturing.

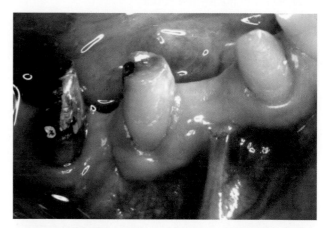

Fig. 3.42 Following healing, adequate bands of attached keratinized tissue are noted on the buccal aspects of all abutment teeth.

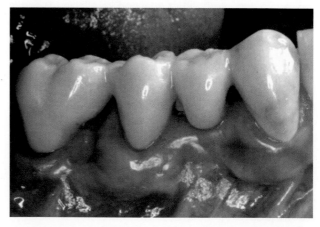

Fig. 3.43 The area has been provisionalized. Note the flat emergence profile of the provisional restoration as it leaves the gingiva in the treated furcation area.

interrupted silk sutures (Fig. 3.40). A lingual view demonstrates the crestal anticipation which was carried out prior to lingual flap suturing, as previously described (Fig. 3.41). Following appropriate healing, no probing depths in excess of 3 mm are present, and adequate bands of attached keratinized tissue are evident on all abutment teeth (Fig. 3.42). A provisional fixed restoration is placed after healing has been completed (Fig. 3.43). Note the flat emergence profile of the provisional restoration exiting from the gingiva in the treated furcation area. The provisional restoration contours are then modified to flow gently to the desired occlusal surface. Such an approach helps prevent soft-tissue pileup in the area and greatly aids home-care efforts, thus promoting long-term periodontal health.

It is also imperative that root-resective therapy be carried out appropriately in cases for which it is indicated, if the desired levels of success are to be attained. Attempts at performing such treatment on teeth without distinct roots are obviously contraindicated. Unfortunately, such therapy is still encountered.

CLINICAL EXAMPLE FIVE

A patient presents having undergone extensive therapy with prior practitioners. This treatment included endodontic therapy, root resection on the maxillary first and second molars, and placement of various restorative materials in the area (Fig. 3.44). A radiograph taken at the time of the consultation visit demonstrates the extent of the

restorative material that had been placed between the maxillary molars (Fig. 3.45). Following removal of this excess restorative material, severe buccal defects are evident around the maxillary molars (Fig. 3.46). Due to extensive bone and attachment loss, the teeth are extracted (Fig. 3.47). After discussions with the prior treating practitioners, it became evident that therapy had proceeded as follows:

Endodontic treatment had been carried out on both maxillary molars. Unfortunately, root

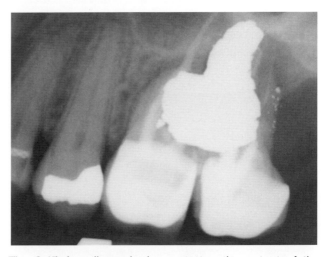

Fig. 3.45 A radiograph demonstrates the extent of the restorative material that has been placed.

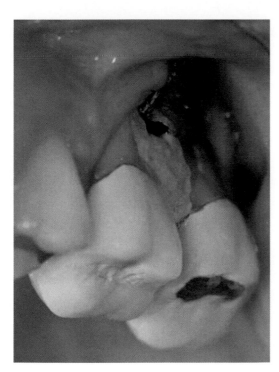

Fig. 3.44 A patient presents with severe periodontal destruction on the buccal aspects of the maxillary first and second molars, and an abundance of restorative material having been placed interproximally in the area.

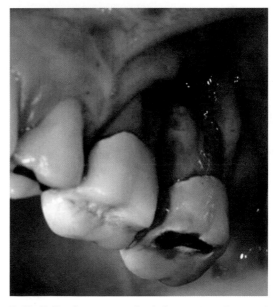

Fig. 3.46 Following removal of the restorative material, severe periodontal destruction is noted in the area.

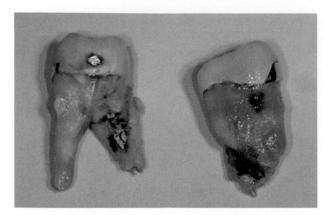

Fig. 3.47 Tooth extraction demonstrates endodontic perforations, and failed attempts at resecting roots that were not individual entities, on both molars.

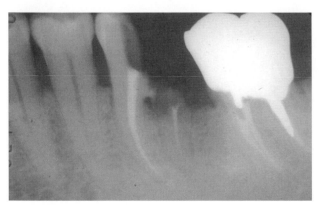

Fig. 3.48 Following hemisection of a mandibular first molar, the distal root has not been removed.

perforations were encountered during both of these endodontic treatments. Attempts were then made to resect the perforated roots from the molars. Because there were not distinct roots (in the case of the second molar, the tooth only had one root), root resection was unsuccessful. The restorative dentist then filled the area with amalgam to "seal off" the attempted root resection. When the patient complained about the aesthetics of the area, the amalgam restorations were covered with white acrylic. The net result of this treatment was the need to remove the teeth, perform regenerative therapy, and subsequently insert implants.

Although not all therapeutic errors are as dramatic as this one, varying degrees of inadequate and incorrect root-resective therapy abound. Such mistakes range from gross failure to remove a resected root (Fig. 3.48), to failure to ensure that

no residual root overhang remains following root resection and extraction (Figs. 3.49–3.54). Fig. 3.49 demonstrates the therapeutic outcome of hemisection of a mandibular first molar and extraction of the mesial root. The distal root was then restored through a full-coverage approach. Unfortunately, a tooth "lip" had been left on the retained distal root. While the restorative dentist placed a crown that fit well on this tooth lip (Fig. 3.49), the area was not conducive to appropriate home-care efforts, as a minifurcation involvement was still present. Three years post-therapy, a severe inflammatory

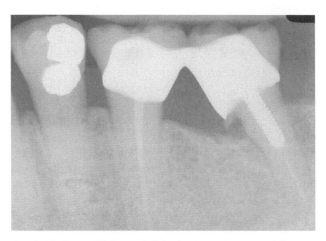

Fig. 3.49 A root "lip" was left in the furcation area following hemisection of the mandibular first molar and extraction of the mesial root. The restoration that has been placed fits well on the root lip. However, the area is not conducive to appropriate home-care efforts.

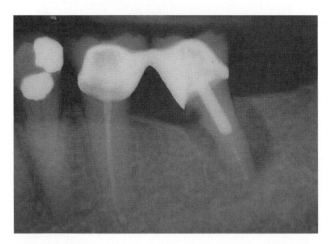

Fig. 3.50 Three years postoperatively, severe periodontal destruction has occurred around the retained distal root of the first molar.

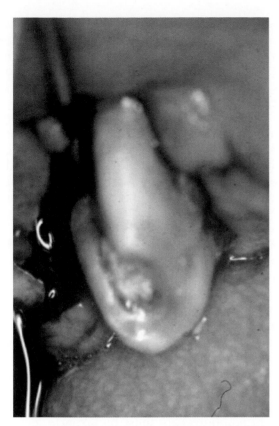

Fig. 3.51 Following root-resective therapy, a root lip was left in the furcation area. The resultant plaque accumulation has led to continued periodontal breakdown in the region.

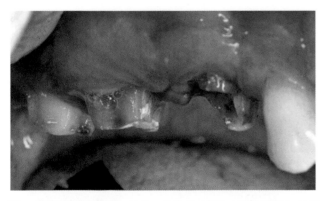

Fig. 3.52 A patient presented having undergone root resective periodontal therapy. Significant pocketing was noted on the buccal aspect of the maxillary first molar.

lesion with extensive osseous loss was noted (Fig. 3.50). The root was subsequently removed.

Retention of such a root lip in the furcation area significantly increases plaque accumulation,

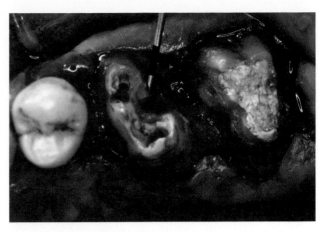

Fig. 3.53 Flap reflection demonstrated a root lip in the root resection area. A deep furcation involvement was present in this region between the two roots. Note the odontoplasty that was successfully carried out to eliminate Class I furcation involvements on the four-rooted maxillary second molar.

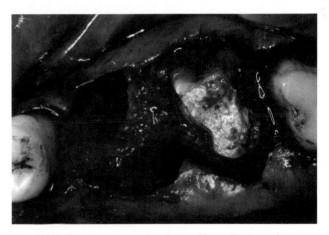

Fig. 3.54 The compromised maxillary first molar was extracted.

hinders home-care efforts, and helps to reinstitute inflammatory periodontal disease in the region. Fig. 3.51 demonstrates the destruction that may occur around such a retained lip.

CLINICAL EXAMPLE SIX

A patient presents having undergone extensive periodontal therapy and tooth provisionalization. Unfortunately, significant pocketing is still evident on the buccal aspect of the maxillary first molar, which had undergone a distobuccal root resection

(Fig. 3.52). Flap reflection demonstrates a root lip where the root resection had been carried out, and a Class II furcation involvement between the retained mesiobuccal and palatal roots of the maxillary first molar (Fig. 3.53). Note that the Class I furcation involvements on the four-rooted maxillary second molar had been successfully treated with odontoplasty. The treatment options now available with regard to the first molar include tooth sectioning and removal of the mesiobuccal root. However, such an approach would not be advantageous, with regard to either stress distribution under function or patient home care. The tooth is therefore extracted (Fig. 3.54). Tooth replacement will now take the form of either a three-unit fixed splint or a single implant.

If the documented levels of predictability are attainable through appropriate root resection, endodontic therapy, and tooth restoration, it is imperative that other treatments to be considered, such as "maintenance", regenerative therapy, or tooth replacement with an implant and crown, at least match these levels of success.

As root resection and endodontic and restorative intervention have become less desirable, due to a lack of facility with the techniques, financial considerations, or both, various regenerative approaches have been championed for treatment of Class II furcation involvements.

Unfortunately, preliminary positive results utilizing either membrane-assisted guided tissue regeneration or other types of grafting and regenerative techniques led some researchers and clinicians to hail a given regenerative approach as a guaranteed means of eliminating Class II furcation involvements. Each approach, in turn, was offered as a method for easily attaining re-attachment and closure of periodontally involved furcations.

As successive products and techniques have fallen short of this claim upon subsequent examination, many clinicians have been all too ready to condemn specific treatment approaches as short-term solutions, at best. The truth undoubtedly lies between the two extremes.

Numerous materials and techniques have demonstrated great promise in regenerating alveolar bone and attachment apparatus in Class II furcation areas. Although each of these approaches requires further study and clinical documentation, they should not be abandoned.

Regardless of which material and approach are utilized to attempt regeneration in a periodontally involved furcation, the following diagnostic and technical modifications to conventional techniques will undoubtedly prove helpful and worthwhile.

All furcations should be debrided with either microscope-assisted instrumentation or rotary burs. Periodontal regeneration in the presence of residual plaque and calculus is highly unpredictable. If all root surfaces bordering a given furcation cannot be accessed for appropriate debridement, regenerative therapy should not be attempted.

Odontoplasty should be performed on all Class II furcations to an extent that would eliminate the horizontal component of a Class I furcation for the tooth in question (Figs. 3.55, 3.56). Decreasing the horizontal component of the involved furcation places a lesser demand on the regenerative procedure to effect furcation closure. This fact is especially important when employing time-sensitive materials such as resorbable membranes, or nonresorbable membranes that must be removed 6–8 weeks after insertion due to plaque accumulation and/or host response.

In addition, care must be taken to ascertain whether or not adequate dimension exists between any restorative margin that is present and the area in which regenerative therapy, including

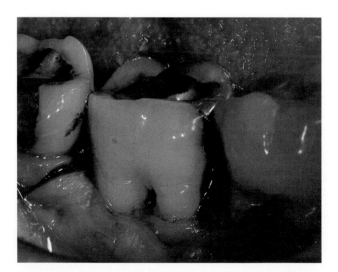

Fig. 3.55 A patient presented with a Class II buccal furcation involvement and a Class III cementoenamel projection on a mandibular second molar. Regenerative therapy was planned in this region.

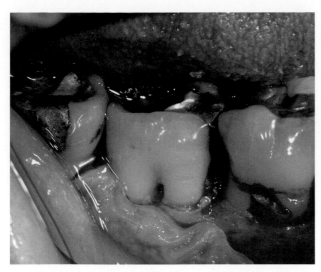

Fig. 3.56 Prior to carrying out regenerative therapy, odontoplasty was performed to eliminate the Class III cementoenamel projection, and reduce the Class II furcation to the extent that odontoplasty would be performed to eliminate a Class I furcation. This step would significantly decrease the horizontal dimension of the residual furcation involvement.

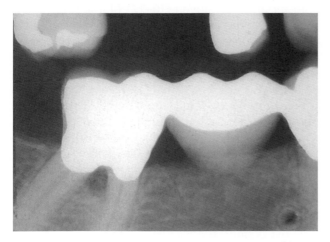

Fig. 3.57 Attempts at regenerative therapy in the Class II buccal furcation involvement of the mandibular second molar would have a limited prognosis due to the position of the restorative margin at the entrance to the furcation.

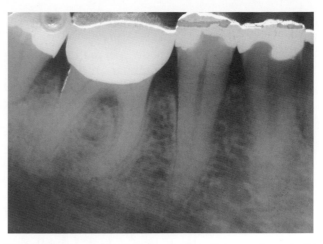

Fig. 3.58 Attempts at regenerative therapy to rebuild damaged alveolar bone and attachment apparatus in the Class II buccal furcation involvement of the first molar should have an excellent prognosis due to favorable interproximal bone height, a short root trunk, and the restorative margin being placed at least 3 mm coronal to the entrance to the furcation.

reattachment, is desired. For example, if a restorative margin has been placed in such a position as to be at the entrance of the furcation, attempts at regenerative therapy in this area are futile. Fig. 3.57 demonstrates such a problem. A Class II furcation involvement is noted on the mandibular second molar, the terminal abutment for a three-unit fixed splint. Unfortunately, the margin of the full-coverage restoration is within 1 mm of the furcation entrance. Attaining periodontal regeneration and reattachment in the face of such violation of the biologic width is not predictable. In contrast, the Class II furcation involvement demonstrated in Fig. 3.58 should prove amenable to regenerative therapy. The levels of the interproximal bone around the tooth are good, and the restorative margin has not been placed in the area in which regeneration is desired.

An in-depth discussion of various materials now being tested and utilized to effect periodontal regeneration in Class II furcations is not the purpose of this text.

Treatment of Class III Furcations

Regenerative therapy performed in Class III furcation involvements is "predictable" but discouraging. Therapy is never predictably successful. To date, no techniques have proven effective in regenerating lost alveolar bone and attachment apparatus, and attaining furcation closure, when treating Class III furcations.

Maxillary vs. Mandibular Furcations

An argument can be made for maintenance of a deeply furcated mandibular molar through continued debridement. In such a situation, if the patient is hesitant to undergo more extensive therapy, including tooth removal, implant placement, and concomitant bone regeneration, attempts at maintaining his or her mandibular molar will result in continued loss of bone buccally and lingually, as the furcation involvement progresses. Even in the face of abscess formation in the furcation area, only the buccal and lingual plates of bone will be damaged. So long as no interproximal periodontal breakdown is noted due to deeper pocketing and/or infrabony defects that may be present, the patient is not ill served in the long term through such tooth maintenance if he or she understands that an ongoing disease process is present, as regeneration can be performed at the time the tooth is eventually removed and an implant subsequently placed.

However, this is not the situation when faced with a deeply furcated maxillary molar. The potential for severe damage to the mesial and distal interproximal bone, and thus to the adjacent teeth, is high should rapid progression of periodontal disease and/or abscess formation occur in the affected maxillary furcation. Due to the positions of the mesial and distal furcations of the maxillary molar, such disease progression will significantly affect supporting bone at the furcation entrances of adjacent teeth. As a result, maintenance of deep furcation involvements on maxillary molars should never be entertained, unless the patient is ill suited for appropriate surgical intervention due to medical considerations, or is of such an advanced age that the risks inherent in tooth retention in such an environment are reasonable.

Selecting the Appropriate Treatment Modality

Prior to developing treatment algorithms and selecting preferred therapeutic modalities, it is incumbent upon the clinician to have a thorough understanding and mastery of the available techniques. In addition to technical competence, the clinician must be well versed in the indications, contraindications, and expected long-term treatment outcomes of each therapeutic approach. The clinician's level of perception will have a significant impact on his or her development of treatment algorithms.

For example, if a patient presents with an endodontic perforation of a maxillary first molar which condemns its mesiobuccal root, available treatment options include root resection and subsequent restoration; tooth removal and replacement with an implant, abutment, and crown; or tooth removal and replacement with a three-unit fixed bridge. Should the clinician believe that, following extraction of an upper molar, the area must be allowed to heal, a subsequent sinus augmentation procedure must be performed and an implant be placed at a third surgical session, it is highly unlikely that such a treatment algorithm would be chosen. However, should the clinician understand that the tooth can be extracted, an implant placed at the time of tooth removal, concomitant regenerative therapy be performed if necessary, and the implant be restored approximately 5 months later, the idea of implant utilization becomes much more attractive. Either of these approaches has demonstrated high rates of long-term success when appropriately employed (10–12) (Table 3.1). Use of one of these treatment modalities would avoid the need to involve the adjacent teeth in a fixed prosthesis. Similarly, if the clinician does not understand how to appropriately perform root-resective techniques, and has had negative experiences when employing such therapies, this treatment option will not be considered.

Conscientious clinicians perform both therapeutic and cost-benefit analyses prior to developing treatment algorithms. The cost-benefit analysis will include both biologic and financial costs to the patient. Once again, the clinician's understanding of therapeutic potentials will significantly impact the cost-benefit analysis.

The greatest biologic cost is undoubtedly paid if a three-unit fixed prosthesis is utilized to replace a compromised maxillary first molar. Nevertheless, this treatment option will be chosen if the clinician is uncomfortable with root-resective techniques and does not understand how to replace the extracted molar with an implant without performing a sinus augmentation procedure.

Failure to understand implant placement at the time of maxillary molar extraction, and the mistaken belief that sinus augmentations must be performed in such sites, will result in a greater financial cost to therapy than either a root-resective approach or tooth extraction with simultaneous implant placement and regeneration, and subsequent restoration.

Similarly, implants may be placed at the time of mandibular molar extraction with concomitant regenerative therapy, and yield high rates of clinical success. The question is not whether to perform such therapy, but rather when to utilize a therapeutic approach entailing tooth extraction, implant placement, regeneration, and subsequent restoration, and when to maintain the furcated tooth in question through appropriate periodontal surgical intervention of a resective and/or regenerative nature and necessary restoration. Although implant therapy is not our topic of discussion, it is imperative that the advantages and disadvantages of such treatment be considered when formulating a comprehensive, interdisciplinary treatment plan, whether it be for a single tooth or in anticipation of full-mouth rehabilitation.

When deciding whether to resect a root and retain a furcated molar, or to extract the tooth and replace it, a number of factors must be carefully weighed. The first group of factors fall under the heading of global patient concerns. These include the health of the patient and the willingness and ability of the patient to perform necessary home-care measures. In addition, the psychological make-up of the patient must be considered. A patient who states that he or she cannot imagine having a tooth removed, and wishes to go to any length to try and maintain the tooth, should be treatment planned for root resection and molar retention if at all feasible. In contrast, a patient who states that he or she wants to go through the quickest, least-involved therapy, and is unwilling to accept potential failure in the future, may be better served through tooth removal and implant placement (14).

The presence or absence of parafunction must be carefully ascertained. While destructive to all teeth and their supporting attachment apparati, parafunction is especially damaging to root-resected molars. These teeth by definition have less root structure than is ideal to support the crown of the tooth under function, and do not have root support beneath all aspects of the crown, as would usually be encountered with an intact tooth. As such, these teeth are more prone to fracture in a parafunctional patient than non-root-resected molars. Parafunctional patients must

be willing to faithfully utilize the appropriate bite appliances.

The patient's willingness to commit to long-term maintenance care must also be carefully assessed. Performing complex therapies on patients who will not perform appropriate home care is ill advised. This is true both with natural teeth and implants. While implants are theoretically less susceptible to the initiation of bone destroying inflammatory lesions, neither treatment should be undertaken without the appropriate patient commitment and cooperation.

Finally, the role of the tooth in the patient's overall treatment plan must be carefully weighed, as will be subsequently discussed.

When considering individual tooth characteristics to determine whether or not a given tooth is a good candidate for root-resective therapy, a variety of factors must be assessed (Table 3.2). These include:

- *The ability to eliminate all pocketing around the tooth following root resection:* If pocket-elimination therapy may not be successfully carried out and residual probing depths in excess of 3 mm will remain following therapy, the tooth is a poor candidate for root resection, endodontic therapy, and subsequent restoration.
- *The attachment levels on the residual root(s):* If the periodontal disease around the tooth has resulted in a significant compromise of the bone and attachment apparatus support of the residual root(s), the tooth is a poor candidate for treatment and maintenance.
- *The ability to eliminate residual furcation involvement(s) following root resection:* If a furcation involvement will remain between two roots of a maxillary molar following resection of the third root, the tooth is a poor candidate for treatment and maintenance. Should a Class I furcation involvement be noted between the two retained roots, it is easily eliminated through odontoplasty. However, if a deeper furcation involvement is noted between the two roots to be retained, the tooth should be removed and replaced.

If ideal endodontic therapy cannot be performed on the residual roots due to canal calcification, root morphology, or other factors, the tooth

Table 3.2. Factors influencing tooth retention.

Individual tooth factors	Resect root and retain tooth	Extract tooth
Can eliminate pockets	Yes	No[1]
Can eliminate residual furcation(s)	Yes	No[1]
Attachment levels on residual root(s)	Acceptable	Compromised[2]
Tooth is restorable.	Yes	No[1]
Can do endodontics	Yes	No[1]
Root trunk length	Short	Long[2]
Quantity of interradicular bone	Broad/adequate	Narrow/questionable[2]
Quality of interradicular bone	Cancellous	Cortical[2]
Residual root anatomy	Thick, straight	Thin, curved[2]
Occlusal status	Within the arch	Terminal tooth[2]
Can eliminate mucogingival problems	Yes	No[1]
Other treatment options	Complex	Simple[2]
Tooth important to new treatment plan	No	Yes[1]

[1]Absolute parameter to extract tooth.
[2]Relative parameter to extract tooth.

must be removed and replaced. This is an absolute contraindication to root resection and tooth retention. Consider these factors:

- *The ability to appropriately restore the tooth:* If ideal restoration of the residual tooth cannot be carried out, including the ability to place restorative margins at levels which are wholly accessible to the patient for home-care efforts, the tooth must be removed and replaced. This is an absolute contraindication to tooth retention.
- *Root trunk length:* While a tooth with a shorter root trunk will demonstrate furcation involvement in the face of periodontal breakdown more rapidly than its counterpart with a longer root trunk, the tooth with the shorter root trunk is more amenable to root-resective procedures than a tooth with a longer root trunk. Following root resection from a tooth with a shorter root trunk, more root structure will remain in bone than when root resection has been carried out on a tooth with a longer root trunk. By the time periodontal destruction has

reached the furcation of a tooth with a longer root trunk, a greater percentage of the overall periodontal support of the tooth has been compromised.

- *The quantity of the interradicular bone:* A tooth with divergent roots, and thus a greater quantity of interradicular bone, is more amenable to root-resective procedures than a tooth with roots in proximity to each other, resulting in a thinner, more labile interradicular bony septum. Such a thin bony septum is more prone to resorption during postsurgery healing.
- *The quality of the interradicular bone:* A patient with thicker interradicular bone demonstrates a greater percentage of cancellous bone, and thus of marrow, than the residual thinner interradicular bone found between two roots which approximate each other. This thicker, more cancellous bone is less labile and prone to resorption as a result of postsurgical inflammation, and offers a greater amount of endothelial and pluripotential mesenchymal cells to help initiate healing of the surgically injured periodontal tissues.

- *Residual root anatomy:* A tooth whose residual roots will be thicker and straighter is a better candidate for root-resective therapy than a tooth whose residual roots will be thinner and more curved. This is due both to the ability of the thicker, straighter roots to better withstand functional forces, and the ease of endodontic therapy on such roots as compared to their thinner, more curved counterparts.
- *Occlusal status of the tooth:* By definition, a tooth that has had a root removed from it has less support to withstand functional and/or parafunctional forces. In addition, the support that is present is not ideally placed beneath the crown of the tooth/restoration, to help dissipate these forces. As such, a maxillary first molar that has had a root removed and is within an arch that has a second molar behind it, presents with a superior long-term prognosis to a maxillary first molar that has had a root removed and is the terminal tooth in the arch, all other factors being equal. In the case of a mandibular molar, root resection results in a restoration that is cantilevered off of the retained root of the mandibular molar. Such a clinical scenario does not present with a favorable long-term prognosis. This consideration has been discussed by Langer (15), in an analysis of his published data documenting failures following root-resective therapy and tooth restoration.
- *The ability to provide adequate attached keratinized tissue around the residual roots:* If at least 3 mm of attached keratinized tissue cannot be established around the residual roots to help withstand inflammatory insult as well as the greater demands placed upon the periodontium by the restorative margin, which will out of necessity approach the gingival margin, the tooth must be removed and replaced. This is an absolute contraindication to root resection and tooth retention.
- *Other treatment options available should the tooth be removed instead of undergoing root-resective therapy:* If the tooth in question is a terminal abutment for a fixed prosthesis, which is stable in all other respects, or a key midabutment in a similar prosthesis, it is often logical to attempt to retain the tooth through root-resective therapy. Removal of the tooth, and thus of the prosthesis, would subject the patient to extensive therapies, including either extension of the prosthesis to include additional teeth, if possible, or placement of multiple implants and their subsequent restoration. In contrast, if the tooth in question is a lone-standing mandibular molar, it is more logical to remove the tooth and place an implant at the time of tooth removal with concomitant regenerative therapy, rather than performing root resection, endodontic therapy, and restoration, and being left with a tooth that is ill suited to withstand functional and/or parafunctional forces over time.
- *The importance of the tooth in a new treatment plan:* If the patient is to undergo significant therapy and if the position of the tooth in question is a key position in the planned restoration/reconstruction, it is more logical to remove the tooth and replace it with an implant than to perform root-resective therapy. Although this approach may at first seem counterintuitive, when developing a new treatment plan that entails significant restorative intervention it is logical to provide the most stable abutments possible at all key locations. A successfully osseointegrated implant is more stable long term, and has less chance of requiring additional therapy in the future, than a root-resected molar in many of these situations.

Failure to appropriately manage furcation involvements prior to final restorative intervention results in significantly compromised treatment outcomes and a less than ideal long-term prognosis.

Conclusions

The continued development of new techniques, and the evolution of our understanding of the potentials and limitations of various therapies over time, afford the conscientious clinician more than adequate information to ascertain when to utilize root-resective or implant and regenerative therapies in the treatment of compromised maxillary and mandibular molars (Flow Chart 3.1). It is incumbent upon us all to employ this knowledge to maximize treatment outcomes in the most efficient and reasonable manner. Our patients deserve no less.

References

1. Becker W, Becker BE, Berg L, et al. New attachment after treatment with root isolation procedures. Report for treated class III and class II furcations and vertical osseous defects. Int J Periodontics Restorative Dent 1998; 8: 8–23.
2. Goldman MJ, Ross IF, Goteiner D. Effect of periodontal therapy on patients maintained for 15 years or longer. A retrospective study. J Periodontol 1986;57;347–53.
3. McFall WT. Tooth loss in 100 treated patients with periodontal disease—a long-term study. J Periodontol 1982;53:539–49.
4. Wood WR, Greco GW, McFall WT, Jr. Tooth loss in patients with moderate periodontitis after treatment and long-term maintenance. J Periodontol 1989;60: 516–20.
5. Hirschfeld L, Wasserman B. A long-term study of tooth loss in 600 treated periodontal patients. J Periodontol 1978;49:225–37.
6. Wang HL, Burgett FG, Shyr Y, et al. The influence of molar furcation involvement and mobility of future clinical periodontal attachment loss. J Periodontol 1994;65:25–29.
7. Fleischer HC, Mellonig JT, Brayer WK, Gray JL, Barnett JD. Scaling and root planning efficacy in multi-rooted teeth. J Periodontol 1989;60: 402–9.
8. Nabers CL, Stalker WH, Esparza D, et al. Tooth loss in 1,535 treated periodontal patients. J Periodontol 1988;59:297–300.
9. Carnevale G, DiFebo G, Tonelli MP, et al. A restorative analysis of perio-prosthetic treatment of molars with interradicular lesions. International Journal of Periodontics and Restorative Dentistry. 1989;11: 189.
10. Carnevale G, Pontoriero R, DiFebo G. Long term effect of root resected therapy in molars. A 10 year longitudinal study. Journal of Clinical Periodontology. 1998;25: 209–14.
11. Basten CH, Ammons WF Jr, Persson R. Long term evaluation of resected molars: A retrospective study. International Journal of Periodontics and Restorative Dentistry. 1996;16: 206–19.
12. Fugazzotto PA. A comparison of the success of root resected molars and molar position in implants in function in a private practice: Results of up to 15 plus years. J Periodontol 2001;72:1113–23.
13. Fugazzotto PA. Implant placement at the time of maxillary molar extraction: Treatment options and reported results. J Periodontol, 2008;79:216–23.
14. Fugazzotto PA. Implant placement at the time of mandibular molar extraction: Description of technique and preliminary results of 341 cases. J Periodontol, 2008;79: 737–47.
15. Langer B. Root resection revisited. Int J Periodontics Restorative Dent 1996;16:200–201.

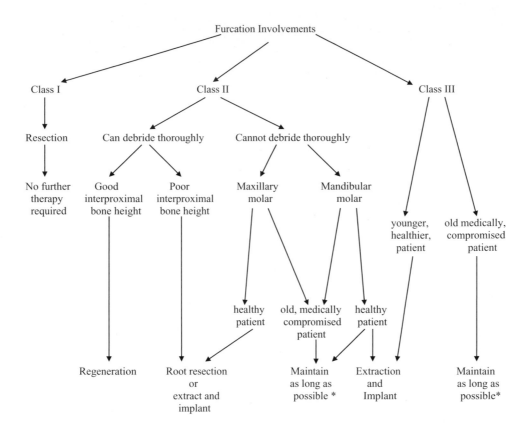

* Patient and clinician must understand risks involved

Flow chart 3.1 Treatment decisions for furcation involvements.

Chapter 4
The Role of Mucogingival Therapy

Paul Fugazzotto

Maximization of treatment results following mucogingival therapy mandates a thorough understanding of the indications, contraindications, and limitations of various therapeutic options, and how best to integrate these options into an individualized, comprehensive treatment plan. Naturally, the need for mucogingival therapy and appropriate definitions of success must first be developed.

The necessity for mucogingival therapy has been a topic of debate in periodontology for a number of decades. Numerous authors have reported upon the ability to maintain periodontal health in the absence of attached keratinized tissues. However, none of these authors has demonstrated periodontal health in the absence of attached keratinized tissues when a restorative margin is present at the gingival crest or intrasulcularly.

A patient presenting with severe gingival recession, a lack of attached keratinized tissue, and an active frenum pull is an obvious candidate for mucogingival therapy to reestablish a stable band of attached keratinized tissue and halt the ongoing disease process (Fig. 4.1). However, it is at least as important to recognize more subtle examples of developing mucogingival problems. A patient who presents with no recession as of yet, a lack of keratinized tissue due to a developmental anomaly which has resulted in mucosa approaching the gingival margin, and a 5–6-mm pocket in the area that is devoid of keratinized tissue, certainly presents with a periodontal milieu that is not conducive to long-term health (Figs. 4.2, 4.3). Whether the soft-tissue margin remains in place and periodontal destruction occurs beneath, or the hard and soft tissues are lost together resulting in a recessive lesion, there is no doubt that such an

area will demonstrate continued periodontal breakdown over time.

It is also important to attain the desired treatment endpoints following mucogingival therapy. Placement of a submarginal soft-tissue autograft, which is separated from residual keratinized tissue by an island of mucosa, does nothing to halt the onset of recession or periodontal disease, until such time as this disease process reaches the submarginal graft that has been placed (Fig. 4.4). Similarly, placement of a "lingerie graft" (Fig. 4.5), which is nothing more than isolated islands of keratinized tissue surrounded by mucosa, serves no functional purpose.

The added demands placed upon the periodontium by the best fitting restorative margins

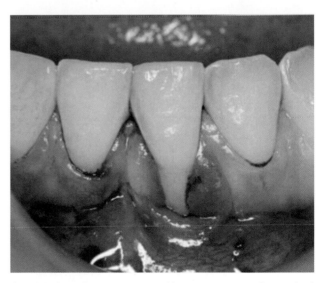

Fig. 4.1 A patient presents with severe recession, a lack of attached keratinized tissue, and an active frenum pull on the buccal aspect of a mandibular central incisor.

Periodontal Restorative Interrelationships: Ensuring Clinical Success, First Edition. Edited by Paul A. Fugazzotto.
© 2011 by John Wiley & Sons, Inc. Published 2011 by John Wiley & Sons, Inc.

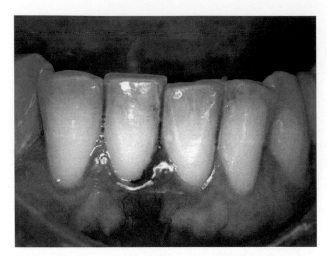

Fig. 4.2 While no active recession is yet noted, the combination of a developmental anomaly characterized by no keratinized tissue on the buccal aspect of the mandibular central incisor and a 6-mm-deep periodontal pocket in this area has resulted in an unstable periodontal milieu. This combination of an osseous defect and a mucogingival problem will continue to break down if not appropriately treated.

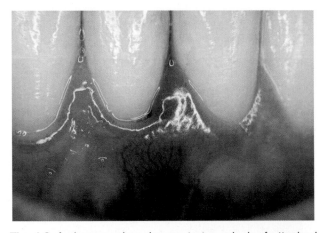

Fig. 4.3 A close-up view demonstrates a lack of attached keratinized tissue and gingival inflammation on the buccal aspect of the mandibular incisor.

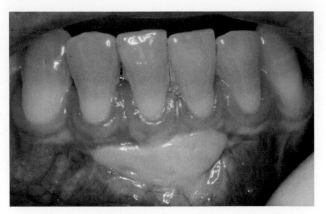

Fig. 4.4 A submarginal gingival autograft has been placed in another patient. Note the mucosa trapped between the preexisting keratinized tissue and the healed graft. This graft offers no assistance in preventing further soft-tissue recession.

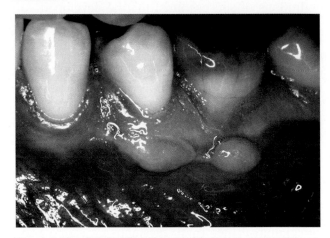

Fig. 4.5 The healed "lingerie graft" demonstrates islands of keratinized tissue surrounded by mucosa. Once again, this therapy offers no benefits to the patient.

mandate the establishment of a stable band of attached keratinized tissue to ensure soft-tissue marginal stability. In the most ideal situation, the attachment apparatus proceeding coronally from the alveolar crest will consist of approximately 1 mm of connective-tissue attachment and approximately 1 mm of junctional epithelial adhesion to the root surface, apical to the gingival sulcus. As a result, a minimum of 3 mm of attached keratinized tissue should be provided to ensure soft-tissue margin stability over time. Such a band of attached keratinized tissue will provide coverage over the alveolar crest, thus helping improve long-term periodontal health and stability. Naturally, any habits (i.e., overaggressive brushing) that contributed to the establishment of recessive lesions must first be identified, discussed, and ameliorated. However, performance of mucogingival therapy after significant recession has already occurred around restorative dentistry, while providing a fiber barrier to help protect against further recession, is a less than ideal treatment philosophy (Fig. 4.6).

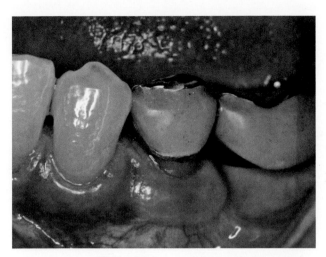

Fig. 4.6 A gingival autograft was placed after significant soft-tissue recession had occurred around the margin of the full-coverage restoration. While this graft will undoubtedly help prevent further recession, timely intervention would have prevented the recession that has occurred.

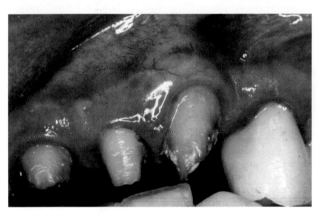

Fig. 4.7 A patient presented having been provisionalized for a full arch reconstruction. The maxillary cuspid demonstrated a lack of attached keratinized tissue. Note also that while an adequate band of attached keratinized tissue was present apico-occlusally on the maxillary lateral incisor, the buccolingual dimension of this tissue was inadequate.

The three-dimensional adequacy of existing keratinized tissues must also be assessed. A patient presented having been provisionalized for a maxillary full-arch reconstruction. A lack of attached keratinized tissue in an apico-occlusal direction was diagnosed on the buccal aspect of the maxillary cuspid. Note that although adequate keratinized tissue is present apico-occlusally on the buccal aspect of the lateral incisor, this tissue is thin buccolingually (Fig. 4.7). In conjunction with gingivo-

plasty procedures around other abutment teeth, a gingival autograft was placed on the buccal aspect of the maxillary cuspid (Fig. 4.8). The provisional restoration was recemented (Fig. 4.9). Following healing and final tooth preparations and buildups, the patient is ready to have the final fixed restorations cemented (Fig. 4.10). An adequate band of attached keratinized tissue is present following augmentation on the buccal aspect of the maxillary cuspid. Twenty-four years after therapy has been completed, the patient presents with maintenance of the soft-tissue contours and height on the buccal aspect of the maxillary cuspid. However, recession has occurred on the buccal aspect of the maxillary lateral incisor, where a buccolingual insufficiency of keratinized tissue had previously been noted (Fig. 4.11). Therefore,

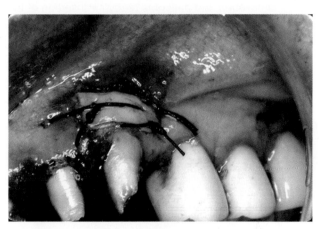

Fig. 4.8 A gingival autograft has been placed on the buccal aspect of the cuspid and secured with interrupted silk sutures, in conjunction with gingivoplasty procedures around the other anterior abutment teeth.

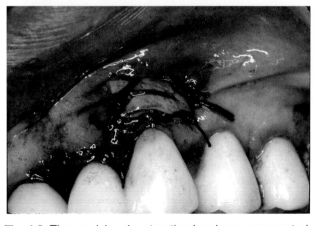

Fig. 4.9 The provisional restoration has been recemented.

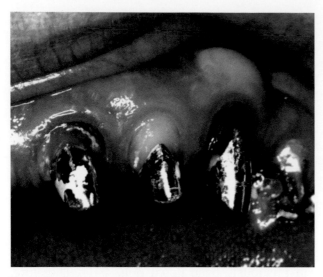

Fig. 4.10 Following soft-tissue healing and tooth preparations and buildups, the patient is ready for insertion of the final maxillary reconstruction. Note the augmented band of attached keratinized tissue on the buccal aspect of the cuspid.

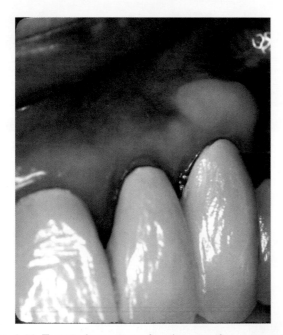

Fig. 4.11 Twenty-four years after therapy, the augmented keratinized tissues on the buccal aspect of the cuspid remain stable. However, soft-tissue recession has occurred on the buccal aspect of the lateral incisor, where the buccolingual dimension of the keratinized tissue was inadequate.

it is imperative that the adequacy of keratinized tissue be assessed in a three-dimensional manner before deciding upon maintenance or another course of treatment.

The buccopalatal dimension of the keratinized tissue must always be considered. A patient who presents with keratinized tissues that are very thin buccolingually, and almost translucent on the buccal aspects of prominent roots, will be at risk upon introduction of a restorative margin near this thin, highly labile soft tissue. The percentage of soft tissue composed of gingival connective tissue is low in such a situation, as most of the bulk is made up of epithelium and rete pegs. As such, this tissue must be augmented prior to placement of restorative dentistry near the gingival margin, regardless of how thick a band of keratinized tissue is present apico-occlusally.

First popularized by Friedman (1–3), augmentation of deficient bands of attached keratinized tissues was championed as a means to prevent the initiation of soft-tissue recession, halt active recession, and provide a "fiber barrier" to help maintain periodontal health over time. Substitution of delicate, friable mucosal tissues, which are characterized by a loose connective tissue, with their denser keratinized counterparts, was championed as a means of withstanding mechanical and inflammatory insult over time, thus protecting the underlying alveolar bone and improving the long-term periodontal prognoses of the teeth (4–9). While such augmentation usually took the form of a gingival autograft harvested from the palate, a variety of pedicle grafts were designed to help eliminate the need for a second surgical site. A comprehensive review of these techniques has been published (10).

Indications for Mucogingival Surgery

These indications include:

- Active recession (11, 12)
- Root sensitivity
- Patient aesthetic dissatisfaction
- Planned restorative margins at the soft-tissue crest or intrasulcularly (13, 14)
- Anticipated orthodontic movement: While many authors have championed the establishment of thick bands of attached keratinized tissue both apico-occlusally and buccolin-

gually in the direction of planned orthodontic movement (15–17), little or no attention has been paid to the need to ensure the presence of adequate bands of attached keratinized tissues around teeth that will have orthodontic movement in the direction opposite to that of the site in question.

If a patient presents with thin bands of attached tissue apico-occlusally or buccolingually on either the buccal or lingual aspects of the teeth, or demonstrates no keratinized tissues in these areas, it is imperative that augmentation of the keratinized tissues be carried out prior to initiation of orthodontic therapy. The combination of the increased plaque accumulation around orthodontic brackets, wires, etc., and the forces the tooth will be placed under, which result in lesions that mimic occlusal trauma histologically, mandates that adequate bands of attached keratinized tissues be present on all aspects of teeth that will undergo orthodontic movement.

CLINICAL EXAMPLE ONE

A patient presents with a cuspid in the position of the maxillary central incisor. This tooth had previously been restored via a full-coverage approach. There is a lack of attached keratinized tissue on the buccal aspect of the tooth (Fig. 4.12). The tooth is provisionalized at the desired gingival level (Fig. 4.13). Note the preparation in the root surface, indicative of the extent of the previous restoration.

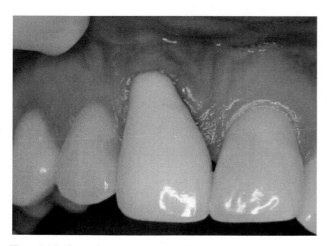

Fig. 4.12 A patient presents with a full-coverage restoration on a cuspid that has erupted in the position of a maxillary lateral incisor. The patient is aesthetically dissatisfied.

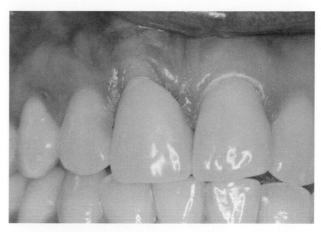

Fig. 4.13 The tooth in the position of the central incisor is provisionalized at the desired final gingival level.

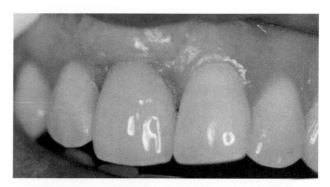

Fig. 4.14 Following odontoplasty to smooth the root surface, placement of a gingival autograft, and tooth restoration following soft-tissue healing, the patient's aesthetic profile has been greatly improved.

Odontoplasty is performed to smooth the root surface, and a gingival autograft is placed (Fig. 4.14). Ideally, a slight gingivoplasty procedure should have been performed following healing to further enhance the aesthetics of the area. However, the patient refused such therapy.

CLINICAL EXAMPLE TWO

A patient in the midst of orthodontic therapy presents with severe recession on the buccal aspect of a mandibular central incisor. Flap reflection and bed preparation demonstrate significant loss of supporting buccal bone (Fig. 4.15). A gingival autograft is harvested from the palate and secured over the area utilizing interrupted silk sutures (Fig. 4.16). Following healing, a thick band of attached keratinized tissue is present in the area (Fig. 4.17). Note the poor color match and contour of the

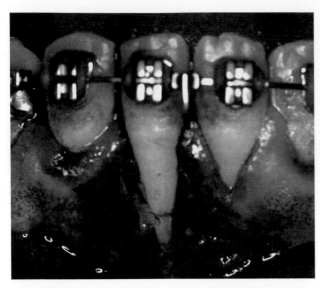

Fig. 4.15 A patient in the midst of orthodontic therapy demonstrates extensive loss of hard tissue on the buccal aspect of the mandibular incisor following bed preparation.

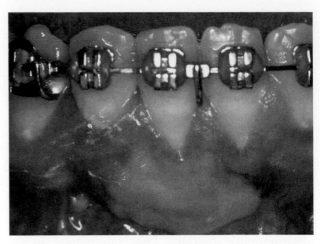

Fig. 4.17 Following healing, a thick band of keratinized tissue is evident on the buccal aspect of the mandibular incisor. Note the problem with gingival contour and color match that was often inherent in such a procedure when performed 25 years ago.

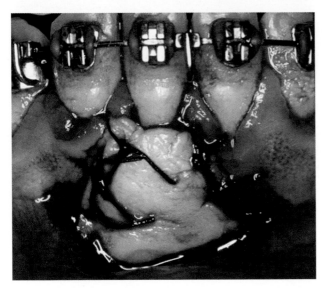

Fig. 4.16 A palatally harvested gingival autograft is placed and secured with interrupted silk sutures.

grafted tissue. Such a nonideal treatment outcome was sometimes encountered when placing gingival autografts in such situations 25 years ago. As will be subsequently discussed, newer techniques are now available, which significantly improve treatment outcomes.

A lack of attached keratinized tissues in the absence of active recession, root sensitivity, or planned restorative or orthodontic therapy is not an indication for mucogingival surgical therapy.

Nonattached Gingival Autografts

The high level of predictability in providing a stable band of attached keratinized tissues through the use of a palatally harvested gingival autograft is well established. The advantages of such a procedure include the ease of procurement of the needed tissues, and the long-term stability of the transplanted and healed tissues (8, 18).

Traditionally, gingival autografts have usually been placed at a level commensurate with the preexisting soft-tissue margins when utilized prior to the development of recessive lesions, and at the bases of recessive lesions when employed to prevent further recession. While such therapy was predictable, the drawbacks of gingival autograft placement included the need for a second surgical site, significant postoperative morbidity at the donor site, and the compromised "color match" between the grafted tissues and their surrounding host counterparts.

CLINICAL EXAMPLE THREE

A patient presents with significant recessive lesions and a lack of attached keratinized tissues on the buccal aspects of the mandibular cuspid and pre-molars (Fig. 4.18). The palatally harvested gingival autograft is placed at the level of the preexisting soft-tissue margins, and secured with 4-0 silk sutures (Fig. 4.19). Two weeks postoperatively, the tissues are healing well. It is evident that an adequate band of attached keratinized tissue will be present following tissue maturation (Fig. 4.20).

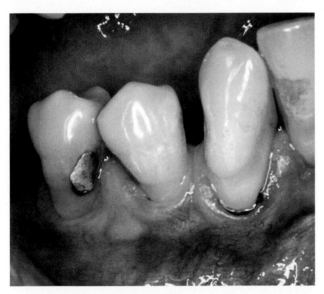

Fig. 4.18 A patient presents with significant recession and a lack of attached keratinized tissues on the buccal aspects of the mandibular cuspid and premolars.

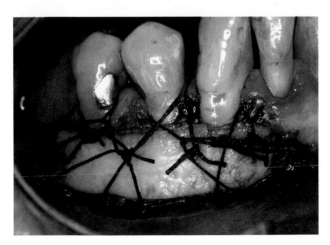

Fig. 4.19 Following appropriate bed preparation, a palatally harvested gingival autograft is placed and secured with silk sutures. Note the bed extension, which has been carried out to ensure that the graft is not "swallowed up" by the surrounding mucosal tissues.

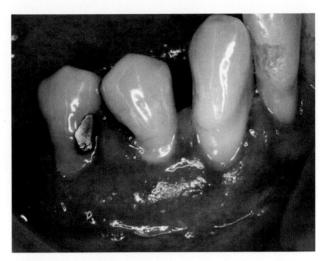

Fig. 4.20 Two weeks postoperatively, excellent soft-tissue healing is noted.

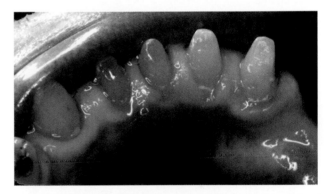

Fig. 4.21 A patient presents with inadequate keratinized tissue on the lingual aspects of the mandibular incisors, which have been provisionalized for full-coverage restorations.

CLINICAL EXAMPLE FOUR

Following tooth preparation and provisionalization, a lack of attached keratinized tissue is evident on the lingual surfaces of the mandibular anterior teeth (Fig. 4.21). A gingival autograft is harvested from the edentulous area next to the mandibular cuspid and secured on the lingual aspects of the teeth following appropriate bed preparation with 4-0 silk sutures (Fig. 4.22). It is crucial that the recipient bed be adequately extended to avoid disruption of the graft through movement of the tongue and its attachments. This is accomplished with a #15 blade and a Golden-Fox 7 knife. Preparation techniques for the recipient bed prior

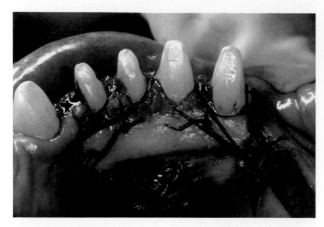

Fig. 4.22 A gingival autograft is harvested from the tissues adjacent to the mandibular anterior teeth and secured with 4-0 silk sutures, following appropriate bed preparation. Such bed preparation is imperative to avoid graft dislodgement due to movement of the tongue and its attachments.

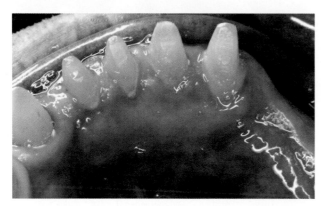

Fig. 4.23 Following healing, a significantly augmented band of attached keratinized tissue is evident on the lingual aspects of the mandibular anterior teeth.

to placement of a gingival autograft on the buccal aspects of teeth will be subsequently discussed. Following healing, an adequate band of attached keratinized tissue is present on the lingual aspects of the mandibular anterior teeth (Fig. 4.23).

The introduction of surgical modifications and refinements afforded the opportunity to effectively cover previously exposed root surfaces with detached gingival autografts. However, such root coverage does not predictably result in reestablishment of true connective-tissue attachment between the augmented soft tissues and the previously exposed root surfaces. The ability of periodontal

ligament cells to migrate over previously exposed root surfaces following gingival autograft placement, in competition with down growth of epithelial cells, has been shown to be approximately 1 mm in all directions. Healing following gingival autograft placement over significant dehiscence defects will therefore result in an area devoid of true connective-tissue attachment of the covering graft to the root surface. The net result is either unattached connective-tissue fibers running parallel to the root surface, or the presence of a junctional epithelial adhesion between the graft and the previously exposed root surface. Either histological outcome is more susceptible to periodontal breakdown and repocketing in the face of inflammation than connective-tissue attachment into root cementum (Fig. 4.24).

As a result, the utilization of gingival autografts to effect root coverage represents a potential compromise, especially in areas that present challenges to appropriate home-care efforts, or where restorative margins are to be placed at the newly established soft-tissue margins or intrasulcularly. A variety of surface preparations has been employed in an effort to attain fiber insertion and reestablishment of connective-tissue attachment between the gingival autograft and previously exposed root surfaces (19, 20–23). Neither citric acid nor other such

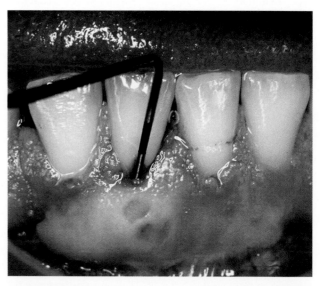

Fig. 4.24 Extensive root coverage had been accomplished through placement of a gingival autograft 6 years ago. Unfortunately, the unattached soft tissues covering the root have repocketed and demonstrate significant periodontal inflammation.

materials, used alone or in conjunction with hand or rotary instrumentation, has demonstrated predictable establishment of such new attachment.

Recent histologic data have demonstrated the ability to help effect connective-tissue attachment through root-coverage procedures by first treating root surfaces appropriately with PrefGel (EDTA) and Emdogain (porcine enamel matrix protein). Prior to graft placement, the exposed root surface is rinsed with sterile water or saline and air dried. PrefGel is applied for 60 seconds. The surface is once more rinsed with sterile water or saline and air dried. Emdogain is applied to the root surface. The soft-tissue graft is then placed over the root surface.

INCISION DESIGNS I

A split-thickness bed is made in the soft tissues apical to the recession around the tooth to be augmented, as well as into the interproximal areas of the adjacent teeth. This bed is made by first extending two vertical releasing incisions at the most distant points of the adjacent interproximal areas from the tooth to undergo soft-tissue augmentation. These vertical incisions are connected at their most coronal extent at the mucogingival junction. In the case of a recessive lesion, they are connected at the level of the mucogingival junction in the interproximal area. This tissue is now reflected and removed in a split-thickness manner to the most apical extent of the releasing incisions. A 15 blade is utilized to bevel all remaining keratinized tissue coronal to the horizontal incision that has been made at the mucogingival junction. Such beveling offers a number of advantages. Beveling of these soft tissues provides a bleeding connective-tissue surface upon which the gingival graft can be overlaid, thus increasing its initial blood supply. In addition, the aforementioned beveling ensures that, following epithelium migration over the grafted tissue onto the host tissues, a smooth confluence of tissues will result, helping to mask the initial incision line. Prior to graft placement, the most apical extent of the bed is extended in a split-thickness manner, utilizing a Golden-Fox 7 knife. This bed is extended laterally 3–4mm at each of its apical corners. Such extension is important to ensure that the apical borders of the graft are not swallowed up by the vestibular soft tissues during healing (Figs. 4.25–4.28).

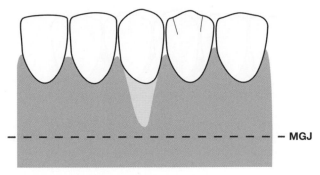

Fig. 4.25 A diagrammatic preoperative view of a mandibular anterior tooth presenting with significant recession. MGJ = mucogingival junction.

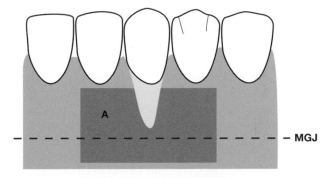

Fig. 4.26 A split-thickness mucoperiosteal bed is created, which extends one tooth mesial and distal to the recessive lesion. A = the prepared mucoperiosteal bed; MGJ = mucogingival junction.

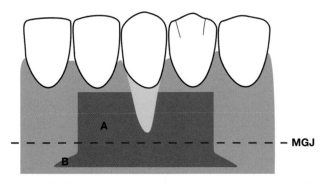

Fig. 4.27 The apical extent of the mucoperiosteal bed is extended mesially and distally with horizontal releasing incisions and further partial thickness reflection, utilizing a Gowen-Fox 7 knife. A = the prepared mucoperiosteal bed; B = the horizontal extensions of the prepared bed; MGJ = mucogingival junction.

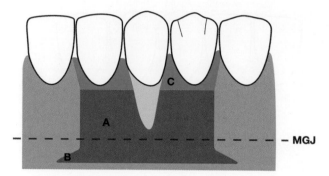

Fig. 4.28 The interproximal soft tissues coronal to the prepared bed are beveled in a split-thickness manner, removing the overlying epithelium. A = the prepared mucoperiosteal bed; B = the horizontal extensions of the prepared bed; C = the beveled tissues coronal to the prepared bed; MGJ = mucogingival junction.

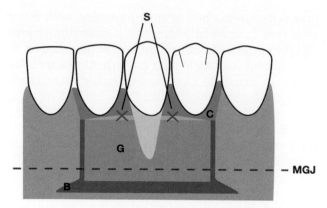

Fig. 4.29 The gingival graft is secured with interrupted resorbable sutures in the interproximal area. B = the horizontal extensions of the prepared bed; C = the beveled tissues coronal to the prepared bed; G = the gingival graft; S = the interrupted sutures; MGJ = mucogingival junction.

The graft is appropriately contoured and placed over the receptor bed. Interrupted gut sutures are utilized to secure the graft at its most coronal extent in the interproximal areas (Fig. 4.29). No other sutures are placed. The lip is manipulated to ensure that adequate apical bed extension has been carried out, both to avoid displacement of the apical border of the graft and to ensure that the apical border of the graft will not be lost beneath the vestibular mucosa during healing.

Lateral Pedicle Flaps

Lateral pedicle flaps have been utilized both to establish bands of keratinized tissue and to cover exposed root surfaces (24–30). The potential advantages of such an approach are the elimination of a second surgical site and a color match superior to that of a detached gingival autograft. A limitation of pedicle flap surgery is the need for an adequate amount of keratinized tissue lateral to the site to be treated for performance of a pedicle flap. Clinicians have previously advocated placing a palatally harvested, detached gingival autograft lateral to the root to be covered, to establish an adequate band of attached keratinized tissue for use in a pedicle graft to effect root coverage. The rationale behind such a procedure is that by rotating a pedicle graft to effect root coverage rather than placing a gingival autograft over a denuded root, the success rate of root coverage is higher due to the maintenance of a blood supply

to the pedicle graft. The drawbacks to such an approach include the need to palatally harvest tissue, and the aforementioned problem of color match of the placed gingival autograft with the adjacent tissues.

CLINICAL EXAMPLE FIVE

A patient presents with significant recession and a lack of attached keratinized tissue on the buccal aspect of the mandibular cuspid. The premolar also requires augmentation of the inadequate band of attached keratinized tissue on its buccal surface (Fig. 4.30). Inadequate keratinized tissue is present distal to the cuspid for rotation as a pedicle graft. A gingival autograft is therefore harvested from the palate (Fig. 4.31). Microfibrillar collagen is placed over the donor site prior to utilization of periodontal dressing, to help control hemostasis (Fig. 4.32). A recipient bed is prepared to accept the gingival autograft on the buccal aspect of the mandibular premolar, as previously described (Fig. 4.33). The gingival graft is secured on the buccal aspect of the premolar utilizing interrupted gut sutures (Fig. 4.34).

Following healing, the augmented band of keratinized tissue on the buccal aspect of the premolar now affords more than adequate tissue for rotation as a pedicle flap over the recessive lesion on the buccal aspect of the cuspid (Fig. 4.35). An incision is made around the recessive lesion on the cuspid with a 15 blade (Fig. 4.36). This incision is of such an extent as to eliminate unattached soft

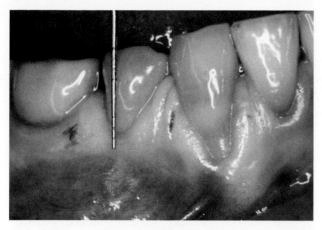

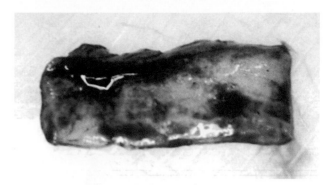

Fig. 4.31 A gingival autograft is harvested.

Fig. 4.30 A patient presents with significant recession and a lack of attached keratinized tissue on the buccal aspect of the mandibular cuspid, and inadequate attached keratinized tissue on the buccal aspect of the mandibular premolar.

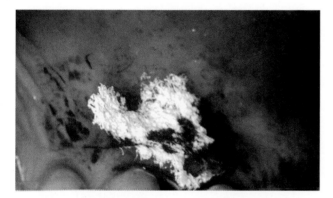

Fig. 4.32 Microfibrillar collagen is placed over the donor site prior to application of periodontal packing to help control hemostasis.

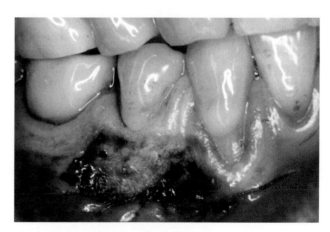

Fig. 4.33 A recipient bed is prepared on the buccal aspect of the mandibular premolar.

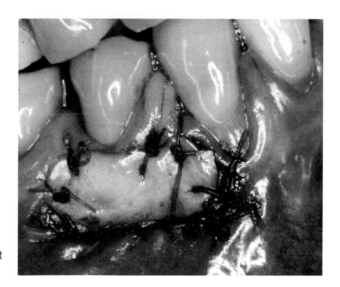

Fig. 4.34 The gingival autograft is secured with interrupted gut sutures.

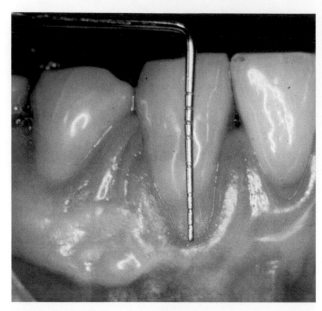

Fig. 4.35 Following soft-tissue healing, the attached keratinized tissue on the buccal aspect of the premolar has been significantly augmented. Adequate tissue is now present for rotation as a pedicle graft to cover the exposed cuspid root.

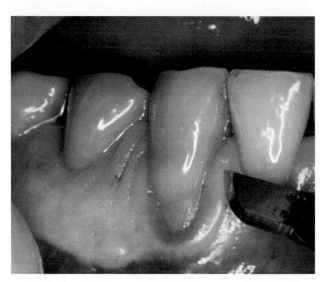

Fig. 4.36 An initial incision is made along the periphery of the recessive lesion on the cuspid.

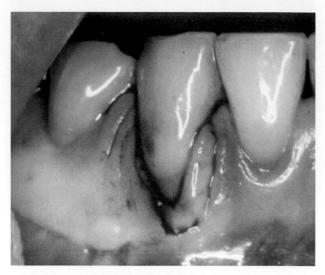

Fig. 4.37 The incision has been made so as to remove all unattached soft tissues surrounding the recessive lesion.

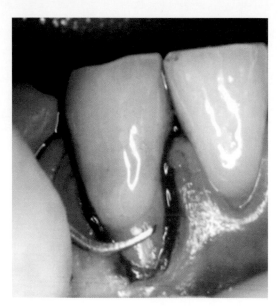

Fig. 4.38 The exposed root is meticulously root planed.

tissue from around the borders of the recession (Fig. 4.37). Following removal of this tissue, the root is meticulously root planed (Fig. 4.38). A vertical releasing incision is now made on the side of the recessive lesion farthest from where the pedicle flap will be rotated (Fig. 4.39). A submarginal incision is outlined on the buccal aspect of the premolar and connects to a distal vertical releasing incision, which in turn connects at its most apical extent to a cut-back releasing incision, toward the direction in which the pedicle flap will be rotated. Finally, a mucogingival flap is reflected in a split-thickness manner, leaving periosteum and some connective tissue intact over the buccal aspect of the premolar (Fig. 4.40). The pedicle flap is rotated over the recession lesion of the cuspid and secured

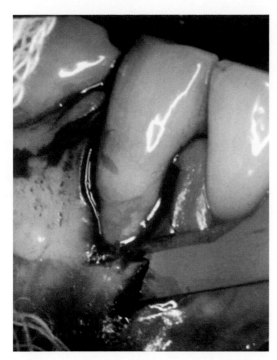

Fig. 4.39 An initial vertical incision is made on the aspect of the recessive lesion farthest from the pedicle graft, which will be rotated.

with interrupted gut sutures, as will be subsequently described (Fig. 4.41). The fact that a split-thickness dissection was performed over the premolar will help ensure that, following healing, an adequate band of attached keratinized tissue will remain in this area. Subsequent to final healing, the augmented band of keratinized tissue is evident over both the premolar and the previously recessed cuspid (Fig. 4.42).

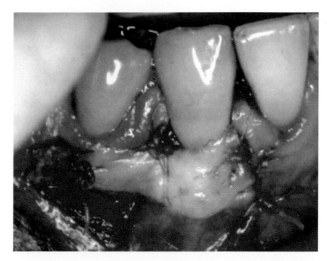

Fig. 4.41 A pedicle flap is rotated over the recession lesion on the cuspid and secured with interrupted gut sutures.

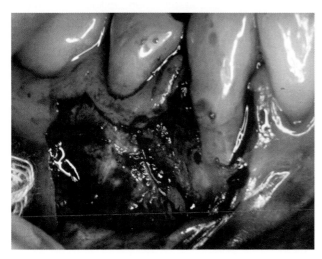

Fig. 4.40 A horizontal incision extends from the recessive lesion submarginally past the premolar. A vertical releasing incision extends from the distal aspect of the premolar and is connected to a cut-back releasing incision at its most apical extent. A split-thickness flap reflection is carried out, leaving periosteum and connective tissue covering the bone on the buccal aspect of the premolar.

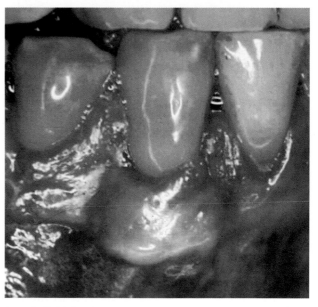

Fig. 4.42 Following soft-tissue healing, coverage of the previously exposed root surface of the cuspid by keratinized tissue is evident. Adequate attached keratinized tissue is also present on the buccal aspect of the premolar.

Lateral pedicle flaps have been performed to effect root coverage both with and without citric acid root treatment. No studies have demonstrated predictable histologic new attachment of the pedicle flap to the previously exposed root surface, either in the presence or absence of citric acid root treatment. As a result, the aforementioned histologic compromise of a junctional epithelial adhesion to the root surface also exists following conventional pedicle-flap therapy. PrefGel and Emdogain use, as described in conjunction with detached gingival autograft placement, should be utilized with pedicle grafts to help effect true connective-tissues attachment of the covering tissues to the previously exposed root surface.

INCISION DESIGN II

A 15 blade is utilized to excise the tissues along the border of the recessive lesion. These tissues are removed with a curette, and care is taken to ensure that the periodontal ligament surrounding the recessive lesion has been reached. The incision is carried beyond the mucogingival junction on the side of the recessive lesion farthest from the site where the pedicle graft will be rotated. For example, if the pedicle graft will come from tissues distal to the recessive lesion, an incision on the mesial aspect of the recessive lesion is extended approximately 4 mm beyond the mucogingival junction. A subsulcular incision is now made extending from the initial incision on the side of the recessive lesion closest to where the pedicle will be rotated, and carried two teeth distal to the recessive lesion. This horizontal incision stops in the interproximal papilla distal to the tooth two teeth away from the recessive lesion, at its most distal aspect. A vertical releasing incision is now made from this most distal extent of the horizontal releasing incision, approximately 4 mm beyond the mucogingival junction. A 45-degree angled cut-back incision is made from the most apical extent of the vertical releasing incision toward the tooth with the recessive lesion (i.e., toward the direction in which the pedicle will be rotated; Figs. 4.43–4.47).

The tissues on the buccal aspects of the two teeth distal to the recessive lesion are now reflected in a split-thickness manner. If the keratinized aspect of this mucoperiosteal flap is at least 2 mm in thickness buccolingually, the pedicle flap is

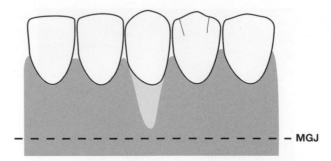

Fig. 4.43 A diagrammatic representation of a mandibular anterior tooth that demonstrates significant recession. MGJ = mucogingival junction.

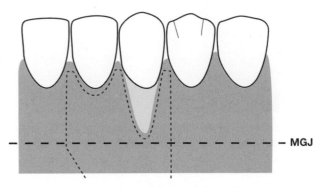

Fig. 4.44 A diagrammatic representation of the flap design employed for rotation of a pedicle flap toward the recessive lesion. Note that the horizontal incisions do not reach the peaks of the interproximal soft-tissue papillae. MGJ = mucogingival junction.

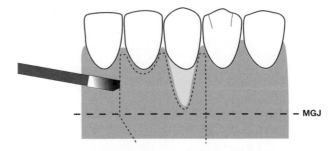

Fig. 4.45 All vertical incisions are made in a beveled manner. MGJ = mucogingival junction.

rotated toward the recessive lesion until its most mesial aspect meets the incision which has been placed on the side of the recessive lesion most distant from the pedicle area.

The flap is now sutured as follows: A suture engages the pedicle flap where it approximates the

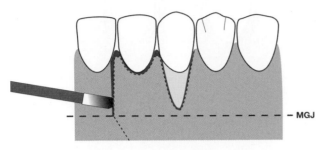

Fig. 4.46 The incision bevels toward the radicular surface of the adjacent tooth, slightly away from the line angle of the tooth. MGJ = mucogingival junction.

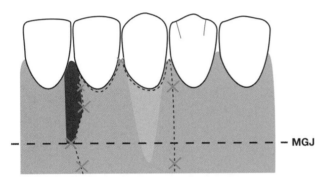

Fig. 4.47 Following a split-thickness reflection, the pedicle flap is rotated over the recessive lesion, having been greatly facilitated by the apical cut-back incision, which is made at the site from which the pedicle is moved. X = interrupted sutures; MGJ = mucogingival junction.

soft tissues on the most distant aspect of the recessive lesion, in the coronal one-third of the incision. An interrupted suture is tied as previously described. A second interrupted suture is placed in the apical one-third of this incision, once again securing the pedicle flap to fixed tissues on the most distant aspect of the recessive lesion. The vertical releasing incision on the pedicle flap farthest from the recessive lesion is now secured with an interrupted suture at its midpoint. A second interrupted suture is utilized to secure this vertical releasing incision in its crestal one-third. Two interrupted sutures are utilized to secure the cut-back incision.

If the buccolingual thickness of the keratinized tissues of the mucoperiosteal flap is less than 2 mm, a connective-tissue graft is first secured over the recessive lesion with interrupted sutures, in the manner previously described for securing a detached gingival autograft. The pedicle flap is then rotated and secured over the recessive

lesion and the connective-tissue graft, as described above.

Connective-Tissue Grafts

The use of connective-tissue grafts beneath coronally positioned flaps has been advocated as a means of attaining root coverage while lessening the trauma of the secondary surgical site and affording a superior color match between the grafted area and the adjacent soft tissues (31–36). Rather than harvesting palatal tissues through an external incision, resulting in an exposed, often painful site that must heal through a large area of secondary intention, a palatal flap is reflected, a connective-tissue graft is harvested from beneath the flap, and the flap is sutured in its original position. The net result is a markedly reduced area that requires secondary intention healing, a much less eventful postoperative course, and decreased postoperative discomfort for the patient. The graft is placed beneath a split-thickness coronally positioned flap in the area where root coverage is desired. The repositioning of such a flap ensures a superior color match and aesthetic outcome, when compared to conventional gingival autograft placement (Fig. 4.48–4.53).

Despite the advantages of this approach, new attachment between the previously exposed root surface and the connective-tissue autograft has not been predictably demonstrated. Final healing is characterized by either a space between parallel running connective-tissue fibers and the root surface, or the interposition of a long junctional epithelial adhesion (37–40). Once again, PrefGel and Emdogain are utilized to help attain true

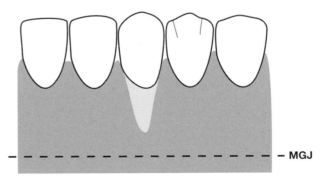

Fig. 4.48 A diagrammatic preoperative view of a mandibular anterior tooth demonstrates significant recession.

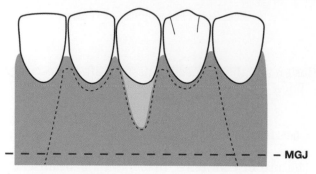

Fig. 4.49 An outline of the incision design for a coronally positioned mucoperiosteal flap. Note that the incision does not reach the soft-tissue peaks of the interproximal papillae, and that the flap extends 1.5 teeth mesial and distal to the recessive lesion. MGJ = mucogingival junction.

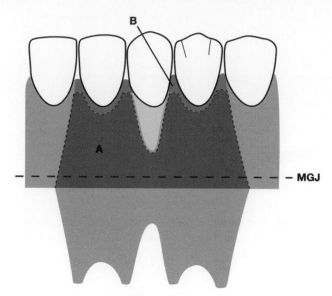

Fig. 4.51 The soft tissues coronal to the prepared bed are beveled in a split-thickness manner, so as to remove all epithelium in the area. B = the beveled papillary soft tissues.

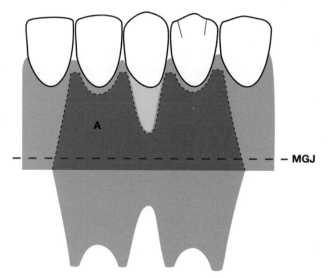

Fig. 4.50 The buccal mucoperiosteal flap is reflected in a split-thickness manner. A = the periosteal bed created through a split-thickness approach.

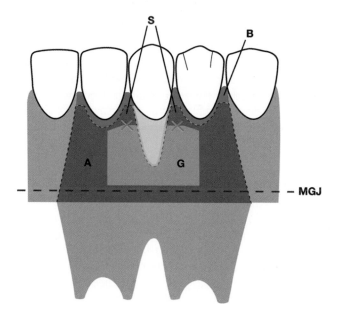

Fig. 4.52 A connective tissue gingival graft is positioned over the recessive lesion and secured with interrupted resorbable sutures. G = the connective tissue graft; S = the interrupted sutures.

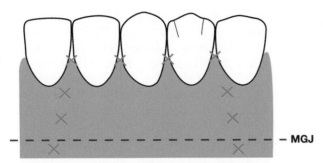

Fig. 4.53 The buccal mucoperiosteal flap is coronally positioned and sutured with interrupted sutures. The interrupted sutures are first placed in the interproximal areas. Interrupted sutures are then used to close the mesial and distal releasing incisions.

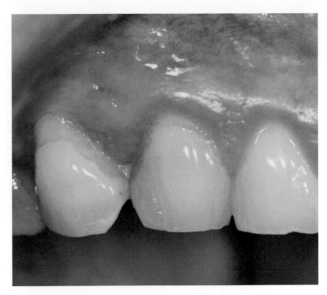

Fig. 4.55 Following placement of a connective tissue autograft beneath a coronally positioned flap and subsequent soft-tissue healing, the previously exposed root surfaces are covered, and the apico-occlusal and buccolingual dimensions of the keratinized tissues in the area are significantly augmented.

covering flap were secured with interrupted gut sutures. Following healing, complete root coverage has been attained, and the thickness of keratinized tissue both apico-occlusally and buccolingually has been significantly increased (Fig. 4.55).

Guided Tissue Regeneration

The use of resorbable or nonresorbable occluding membranes to exclude epithelial cells from a healing periodontal defect, thus allowing migration of slower moving periodontal ligament cells over previously exposed root surfaces and resulting in reestablishment of true connective-tissue fiber insertion into the root, has been well documented. While initially utilized in the treatment of infrabony osseous defect or furcation involvements that were not amenable to resection and elimination, guided tissue regeneration (GTR) therapy has also been applied to the treatment of root-surface dehiscences (44–51). A variety of resorbable and nonresorbable membranes has been utilized to effect such therapy, with and without mechanical or rotary root-surface preparation. The predictability of such treatment in attaining coverage of previously exposed root surfaces has been reported

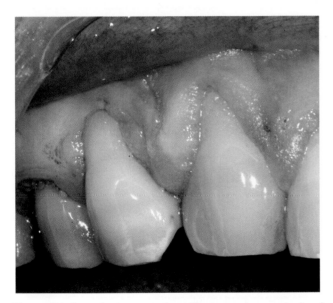

Fig. 4.54 A patient presents with recession, a lack of attached keratinized tissue, and aesthetic dissatisfaction on the buccal aspects of the maxillary cuspid and premolar.

attachment of the graft to the previously exposed root surface.

CLINICAL EXAMPLE SIX

A patient presents with active recession and a lack of attached keratinized tissues on the buccal aspects of the maxillary right cuspid and first premolar (Fig. 4.54). A connective-tissue graft is harvested from the palate and placed beneath a coronally positioned buccal mucoperiosteal flap. First the connective-tissue graft and then the as equal to connective-tissue graft placement beneath coronally positioned flaps. The potential advantage of GTR therapy over connective-tissue graft placement in such a situation is the redevelopment of connective-tissue fiber insertion into the root surface, as compared to the long junctional epithelium or parallel running connective-tissue fibers which result following connective-tissue graft placement over exposed root surfaces (52–60). The disadvantages to the utilization of GTR therapy in the treatment of root-surface dehiscences are the added material expense, the second surgical visit to remove a nonresorbable membrane if one is utilized, and the frequent need for secondary gingivoplastic procedures to effect an acceptable aesthetic outcome.

Indications for Emdogain Use

Porcine enamel matrix proteins are harvested, carefully selected, processed, and packaged under the trade name Emdogain. Emdogain has demonstrated the ability to effect cementogenesis, bone regeneration, and development of connective-tissue fiber insertion between the regenerated bone and cementum in the treatment of infrabony defects (61–84).

The successful utilization of PrefGel and Emdogain in the treatment of infrabony and furcation defects, when appropriately applied, has led to its utilization in the treatment of exposed root surfaces (85–91). Following mechanical and/or rotary debridement, the PrefGel and Emdogain are applied as previously described, and a coronally positioned flap is sutured into place. The result is predictable root coverage and enhanced establishment of reattachment of the connective tissues of the coronally positioned flap to the previously exposed root surfaces (92–97).

INCISION DESIGN III

A sulcular incision is made in the area of recession. This sulcular incision is carried subsulcularly as it approaches the interproximal papillae, and is extended one tooth mesial and distal of the tooth with the recessive lesion. Vertical releasing incisions are placed, connecting to the subsulcular horizontal incisions in the papillae one tooth removed on either side from the tooth with the recessive lesion. These vertical releasing incisions

are carried past the mucogingival junction approximately 4 mm. A mucoperiosteal flap is reflected in a partial thickness manner. The residual soft tissues in the papillary areas from which the flap is reflected are beveled, as previously described (Figs. 4.56–4.60). The advantages of such beveling have already been elucidated. The periodontal ligament area bordering the recessive lesion is curetted, so as to remove all residual epithelium, and to open up the periodontal ligament and thus better access the pluripotential cells in the periodontal ligament to contribute to healing and reattachment (Fig. 4.60). The measurement from the point of desired root coverage to the bone crest in the recessive lesion area is x. The measurement from the bone crest at the base of the recessive lesion to the mucogingival junction is y. If y is $\geq x + 3$, no connective-tissue graft will be placed prior to root treatment and flap advancement. However, if $y < x + 3$, a connective-tissue graft will be placed and secured with interrupted sutures as

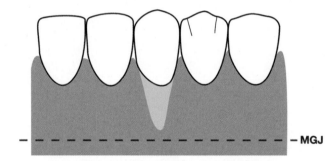

Fig. 4.56 A diagrammatic representation of a mandibular anterior tooth demonstrating significant recession. MGJ = the mucogingival junction.

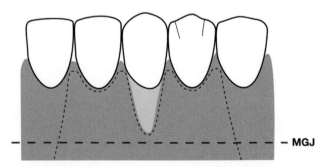

Fig. 4.57 An outline of the incision design for a coronally positioned mucoperiosteal flap. Note that the incision does not reach the soft-tissue peaks of the interproximal papillae, and that the flap extends 1.5 teeth mesial and distal to the recessive lesion. MGJ = mucogingival junction.

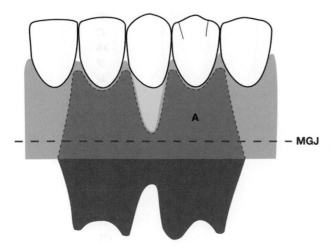

Fig. 4.58 The buccal mucoperiosteal flap is reflected in a split-thickness manner. A = the periosteal bed created through a split-thickness approach.

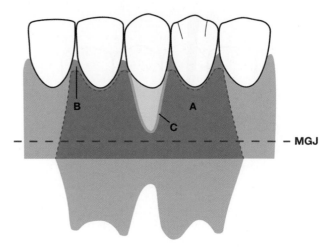

Fig. 4.60 The periodontal ligament surrounding the recessive lesion is curetted, so as to open up the ligament space and better access the pluripotential mesenchymal cells that are present. C = the curetted periodontal ligament space.

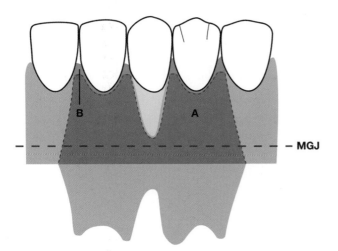

Fig. 4.59 The soft tissues coronal to the prepared bed are beveled in a split-thickness manner so as to remove all epithelium in the area. B = the beveled papillary soft tissues.

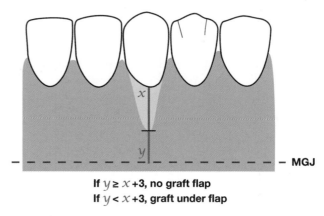

If $y \geq x$ +3, no graft flap
If $y < x$ +3, graft under flap

Fig. 4.61 A measurement is taken to compare the residual keratinized tissue apical to the recessive lesion, and the height of the recessive lesion that must be covered. x = the height of the recessive lesion; y = the residual keratinized tissue apical to the recessive lesion. If $y \geq x + 3$, no connective tissue graft is placed.

previously described, following root treatment and prior to coronal flap repositioning (Fig. 4.61).

The exposed root is debrided with curettes, and treated with PrefGel for 60 seconds. The root surface is rinsed with sterile saline and Emdogain is applied (Figs. 4.62–4.64). The connective-tissue autograft is placed over the exposed root surfaces and secured with resorbable interrupted sutures (Fig. 4.65). If no connective-tissue graft is to be placed, the mucoperiosteal flap is coronally advanced to attain complete coverage of the exposed root surface. If necessary, flap mobility

may be enhanced by adding horizontal releasing incisions at the apical extents of the vertical releasing incisions, and performing additional flap reflection. The flap is secured with interrupted sutures in the interproximal areas. The first two sutures are placed in the interproximal areas between the tooth which has exhibited recession and the adjacent tooth. The next two sutures are placed in the interproximal areas one tooth removed on either side from the tooth exhibiting the recession. The

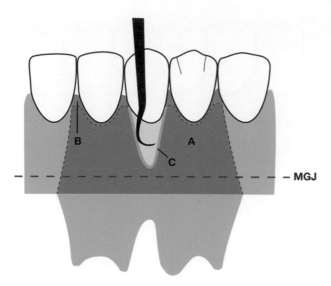

Fig. 4.62 The root surface is curetted.

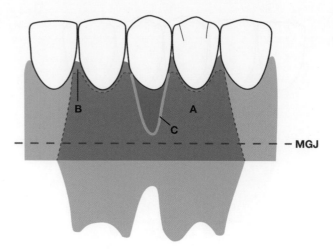

Fig. 4.64 Following rinsing of the root surface with sterile saline, the exposed root surface is covered with porcine-derived enamel matrix protein (Emdogain).

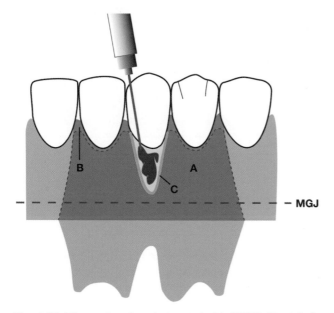

Fig. 4.63 The root surface is treated with EDTA (Pref Gel).

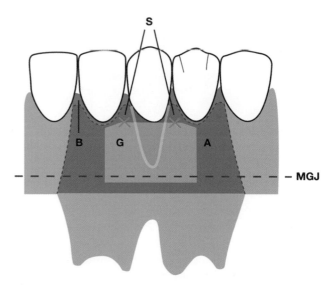

Fig. 4.65 A connective tissue graft is placed over the recessive lesion and secured with resorbable interrupted sutures. G = the connective tissue gingival autograft; S = the interrupted sutures.

vertical releasing incisions are secured. The first suture is placed in the apical one-third of the vertical releasing incision. This suture enters the mucoperiosteal flap, proceeds in a coronal manner, and enters the fixed soft tissues lateral to the releasing incision. The suture is then secured as previously described. It is imperative that this suture extend from the mucoperiosteal flap to the fixed tissues in a coronal manner, so as not to work against attainment of passive coronal flap repositioning. A second suture is now placed in the coronal one-

third of the releasing incision in a similar manner. The second vertical releasing incision is sutured in a manner identical to the first (Fig. 4.66).

As already mentioned, if y > x + 3, a connective-tissue graft is first placed over the exposed root surface and at least 2 mm of bone apical to the recessive lesion, and secured with interrupted resorbable sutures. If an allograft is placed, it is first soaked in PRGF, as discussed below.

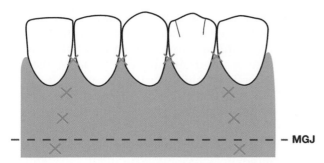

Fig. 4.66 The buccal mucoperiosteal flap is coronally positioned to cover the connective tissue graft. The buccal mucoperiosteal flap is first sutured at each interproximal area with an interrupted suture. The releasing incisions are then closed with interrupted sutures.

The advantages of the above approach include the elimination of a secondary surgical site and the enhanced reestablishment of true connective-tissue attachment to the previously exposed root surface. A disadvantage to this approach is the additional material cost to the procedure. In addition, objective assessment of the treatment endpoints of such therapy demonstrates a potential concern regarding long-term predictability of the newly attained root coverage. By its very existence, the recessive lesion being treated demonstrates the loss of hard and soft tissues over time. It is reasonable to assume that some keratinized tissue would have been present before the recessive lesion began. Therefore, it seems questionable to trust the repositioned soft tissues without their augmentation to provide a thicker, denser tissue, which would be more resistant to mechanical and inflammatory trauma, to maintain their newly attained position over time. If the patient presents with recession and a significant band of attached keratinized tissue at the base of the recession, which is of adequate apical occlusal dimension to allow root coverage and still provide 2 mm of keratinized tissue overlying the buccal alveolar bone, and is at least 2 mm thick buccolingually, there is no need to augment the tissue at the time that a coronally positioned flap is utilized in conjunction with PrefGel and Emdogain to attain root coverage. However, if one or both of these dimensional criteria are not met, a connective-tissue graft should be placed beneath the coronally positioned mucoperiosteal flap at the time of PrefGel and Emdogain use, to ensure adequate postoperative dimensions of keratinized tissue to help prevent redevelopment

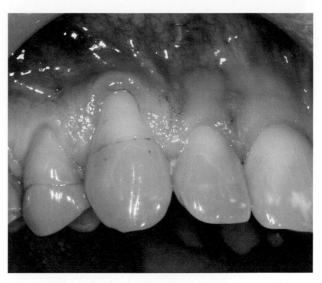

Fig. 4.67 A patient presents with severe recession on the buccal aspects of the maxillary cuspid and premolar, a lack of attached keratinized tissue, and aesthetic dissatisfaction.

of a recessive lesion after introduction of a restorative margin. The allograft tissue comes in varying thicknesses, widths, and lengths; is easy to utilize; and does not require refrigeration or extensive preparation prior to its utilization. Most important, this allograft material has demonstrated the ability to be incorporated well into, and/or replaced by, host connective tissues over time.

CLINICAL EXAMPLE SEVEN

A patient presents with severe recession and a lack of attached keratinized tissues on the buccal aspects of the maxillary cuspid and premolar (Fig. 4.67). Following reflection of a split-thickness mucoperiosteal flap, a connective-tissue allograft is placed and secured with interrupted sutures. The mucoperiosteal flap is then positioned coronally so as to completely cover the graft, and is secured with interrupted gut sutures. Following healing, complete root coverage has been attained, and the apico-occlusal and buccolingual dimensions of the keratinized tissues in the area have been increased (Fig. 4.68).

The use of a soft-tissue allograft beneath a coronally positioned flap at the area of recession has been advocated by a number of practitioners as the means to avoid altogether a secondary surgical site (41–43). However, innovative flap designs

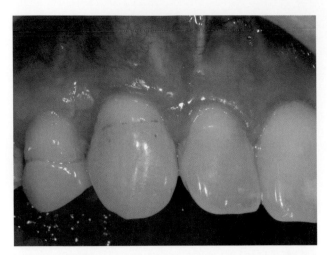

Fig. 4.68 Following placement of a connective tissue allograft beneath a coronally positioned flap and subsequent soft-tissue healing, all exposed root surfaces have been covered, and the keratinized tissues have been augmented in both the apico-occlusal and buccolingual dimensions.

are necessary to ensure complete soft-tissue coverage of the connective-tissue allograft. Failure to do so will result in marked graft resorption. While the appropriate use of such materials demonstrates predictable attainment of root coverage, no studies have as yet documented consistent reestablishment of a connective-tissue attachment between the allograft and the previously exposed root surface.

Constructing a Clinically Based Treatment Decision Tree

To be useful in daily clinical practice, any clinical decision tree must be based upon the unique characteristics of a given patient and the site to be treated. All decision making must be grounded in biologic understanding, supported by literature in refereed journals, and tempered by the realities of technical execution. Manufacturer claims and counterclaims should play no part in the decision making process (Flow Chart 4.1).

TECHNICAL LIMITATIONS

If the use of a coronally positioned flap is to be considered, the execution of such therapy must be predictable. A patient who presents with a paucity

of soft tissue, a shallow vestibule, and severe muscle pull is not a candidate for a coronally positioned flap surgical approach. In addition, should the remaining soft tissues be highly friable, the use of a coronally positioned flap is not indicated. Palatally harvested connective-tissue gingival autografts should be placed in such situations to reestablish stable bands of attached keratinized tissue. A secondary surgical procedure may then be utilized, employing coronally positioned flaps with or without connective-tissue grafts and PrefGel and Emdogain, to effect root coverage if so desired.

WHEN THE RESIDUAL BAND OF KERATINIZED TISSUE IS ADEQUATE

If the apico occlusal dimension of the residual band of keratinized tissue at the base of the recessive defect is at least 2 mm greater than the apico occlusal dimension of the exposed root surface to be covered, and the residual keratinized tissue is at least 2 mm thick buccolingually, the root surface is debrided and treated with PrefGel and Emdogain prior to coronal positioning of the buccal mucoperiosteal flap. The results of this therapy will be enhanced reattachment of the overlying keratinized soft tissue to the previously exposed root surface, as well as establishment of a stable band of attached keratinized tissue to help withstand mechanical and inflammatory insults over time.

WHEN THE RESIDUAL BAND OF KERATINIZED TISSUE IS INADEQUATE

If the apico-occlusal dimension of the residual band of attached keratinized tissue at the base of the recessive defect is not at least 2 mm greater than the apico-occlusal dimension of the exposed root surface to be covered, and/or the buccolingual thickness of the residual keratinized tissue is less than 2 mm, a connective-tissue graft is placed beneath the coronally positioned flap after the exposed root surface has been debrided and treated with PrefGel and Emdogain. The connective-tissue graft must be of sufficient dimension to cover the exposed root surface and overlay the remaining alveolar bone by at least 2 mm. The inclusion of this connective-tissue graft will result in both thicker, more stable keratinized soft tissue over the previously exposed root surface and additional protection of the residual alveolar crest, thus enhancing the stability of both the reestablished soft-tissue margin and the periodontium as a whole.

Mucogingival Therapy at the Time of Crown-Lengthening Surgery

As has been previously discussed, studies that document continued patient health in the face of a lack of attached keratinized tissues are not germane to the discussion of patients requiring crown-lengthening surgery and restorative intervention. None of these studies document continued periodontal health with an absence of attached keratinized tissue in the face of restorative margins at the gingival sulcus or placed intrasulcularly. The increased plaque accumulation which occurs around all restorative margins regardless of the material utilized represents the potential for an increased inflammatory insult to the supporting periodontium. Coupled with the greater lability of mucosal nonkeratinized tissues when compared to attached keratinized tissues in the face of an inflammatory front, it is only logical to establish a stable band of attached keratinized tissue at the time of crown-lengthening osseous surgery, should such tissue not be present.

If the internal connective-tissue wedge removed during thinning of the palatal flap is sufficient in all dimensions, it is always employed when a gingival autograft is to be placed during crown-lengthening osseous surgery. Tissues removed from the distal wedge may be utilized in a similar manner. However, distal-wedge tissues often have to be split and filleted so as to provide an even thickness of tissue, as well to increase the overall graft dimensions. The connective tissue to be utilized should be measured mesiodistally, apical occlusally, and buccolingually to ensure an adequate bulk of soft tissue is present prior to its utilization.

If the necessary quantity of connective tissue cannot be attained from the tissues removed from the internal palatal wedge and/or distal wedge areas, a tissue allograft is employed. This tissue presents with the advantage of affording the clinician a predetermined bulk of soft tissue.

If the clinician has determined in advance of the surgical session that a connective-tissue allograft will be utilized, as should be reasonably expected following a conscientious examination and assessment of the area in question, preparation rich in growth factors (PRGF) is employed in conjunction with the tissue allograft. PRGF is an autogenous plasma product enriched with platelets. Following activation, PRGF releases multiple growth factors and bioactive proteins locally, which modulate wound healing and tissue engineering (98). One of the products obtained through this process is a three-dimensional fibrin scaffold impregnated with growth factors. It has been demonstrated that these growth factors are time released over the first few days of PRGF implantation (99,100). PRGF use accelerates and enhances connective-tissue healing and soft-tissue epithelization.

Prior to placement, a tissue allograft is soaked in the PRGF and the developing fibrin membrane. The net result is an allograft surrounded by a growth factor rich fibrin membrane. This complex is placed beneath the buccal mucoperiosteal flap prior to flap advancement and suturing.

INCISION MODIFICATION

Following completion of osseous resective therapy, the buccal vertical releasing incisions are extended and the split-thickness reflection of the buccal mucoperiosteal flap is carried farther apically, if necessary, to accommodate placement of the soft-tissue graft without hindering final flap repositioning.

The soft-tissue graft must now be secured to the underlying periosteum. Because the more crestal periosteum is no longer in place over the recontoured bone, the soft-tissue graft is secured apical to the site where osseous recontouring has occurred. A suture is placed through the most mesial aspect of the soft-tissue graft, at a position apical enough to engage retained periosteum mesial to the soft-tissue graft. The suture is tied in the manner already described. A similar suture is placed on the distal aspect of the soft-tissue graft, engaging retained periosteum, and tied. The mucoperiosteal flap can now be positioned as desired, through previously described techniques.

An alternative method, which has been advocated in the literature for securing the soft-tissue graft, is to have the suture pass through the buccal mucoperiosteal flap, engage the soft-tissue graft, pass through the soft-tissue graft, reenter the soft-tissue graft from its most internal aspect, pass

Table 4.1. Advantages and disadvantages of various soft-tissue approaches.

Soft-tissue augmentation technique	Advantages	Disadvantages
Nonattached gingival autografts	High level of predictability for increasing band of attached keratinized tissue Easy to procure Can be utilized in areas where muscle pull/shallow vestibule preclude mucoperiosteal flap approach	Significant postoperative morbidity at donor site Concerns with final aesthetics
Connective-tissue autografts	Lesser postoperative morbidity at donor site than conventional gingival autograft	Limitations in size of graft procured
Lateral pedicle flap	No secondary donor site	Must have adequate keratinized tissue lateral to the recessive lesion for rotation
Gingival allograft	No secondary surgical site Size of the connective tissue graft is predetermined.	Adds cost to the procedure Must be completely covered by a mucoperiosteal flap
Guided tissue regeneration	No second surgical site Promotes connective tissue attachment of covering soft tissues to the root surface	Added cost of the procedure Need for secondary procedure if a nonresorbable membrane is utilized Frequent need for secondary gingivoplasty procedures
Emdogain	Promotes attachment of covering soft tissues to the root surfaces	Adds cost to the procedure May have to include a connective tissue graft if inadequate keratinized tissue is present for pedicle rotation or coronal flap repositioning

through the soft-tissue graft, and reengage the buccal mucoperiosteal flap from its internal aspect and pass through the buccal mucoperiosteal flap. The suture is now tied. This procedure is repeated as necessary to secure the soft-tissue graft to the mucoperiosteal flap. The mucoperiosteal flap is then positioned and sutured as previously described. Although this approach may, upon initial examination, appear more advantageous than the approach previously described, this technique does not allow adequate freedom in positioning the buccal mucoperiosteal flap independent of the soft-tissue graft.

Following healing, the net result of treatment will be a thicker dimension of dense connective tissue in all directions, the desired root coverage, and no concerns regarding color match of an onlay graft to adjacent tissues.

Conclusions

The introduction of newer techniques and materials has greatly expanded both the histologic and clinical capabilities of mucogingival surgical therapy (Table 4.1). However, such treatments must be highly individualized and site specific. In addition, success must not be defined by immediate postoperative results, but by long-term stability and predictability under function.

References

1. Friedman N. Mucogingival surgery. Tex Dent J 1957;75: 358–62.
2. Friedman N. Mucogingival surgery: The apically repositioned flap. J Periodontal 1962;3:328–40.

3. Friedman N, Levine HL. Mucogingival surgery: Current status. J Periodontol 1964;35:5–21.
4. Goldman HM. The topography and role of the gingival fibres. J Periodontol Res 1951;30:331–38.
5. Ruben MP. A biologic rationale for gingival reconstruction by grafting procedures. Quintessence Int 1979;11:47–52.
6. Hall WB. The current status of mucogingival problems and their therapy. J Periodontol 1981;52: 556–75.
7. Lang NP, Loe H. The relationship between the width of keratinized gingiva and gingival health. J Periodontal 1972;43:623–27.
8. Matter J. Free gingival grafts for the treatment of gingival recession. A review of some techniques. J Clin Periodontol 1982;9:103–14.
9. Nabers CL. Repositioning the attached gingiva. J Periodontol 1954;25:38–39.
10. Pin Prato G, Clauser C, Cortelini P. Periodontal plastic and mucogingival surgery. Periodontol 2000;9;1995: 90–105.
11. Sullivan HC, Atkins JH. Free autogenous gingival grafts. I. Principles of successful grafting. Periodontics 1968;6:121–29.
12. Hall WB. Gingival augmentation/mucogingival surgery. In: Proceedings of the World Workshop in Clinical Periodontics. Chapter VII. Chicago: American Academy of Periodontology 1989.
13. Nevins R: Attached gingiva: Mucogingival therapy and restorative dentistry. Int J Peridont Restor Dent 1986;6:9–52.
14. Waerhaug J. Tissue reactions around artificial crowns. J Periodontol 1953;54: 172–81.
15. Boyd R. Mucogingival considerations and their relationship to orthodontics. J Periodontol 1978;49: 67–76.
16. Maynard JG. The rationale for mucogingival therapy in the child and adolescent. Int J. Periodontics Restorative Dent 1987;1:37–51.
17. Maynard J G. Mucogingival considerations for the adolescent patient. Volume I. Quintessencance Books, Chicago, p. 291–304
18. Nevins M, Mellonig J T. Periodontal therapy. Clinical applications and evidence of success. Volume I. Quintessencance Books, Chicago, p. 279–90.
19. Miller PD. Root coverage using a free soft tissue autograft following citric acid application. I. Technique. Int J Periodontics Restorative Dent 1982;2:65–70.
20. Babay N, Fugazzotto PA, Ruben MP. Histologic evaluation of soft tissue attachment to acid—enzyme treated root surfaces. Int J Periodontics Restorative Dent 1985;5:77–87.
21. Bertrand PM, Dunlap RM. Coverage of deep wide gingival clefts with free gingival autografts: Root planing with and without citric demineralization. Int J Periodontics Restorative Dent 1988;8:65–77.
22. Ibbot CG, Oles RD, Laverty WH. Effects of citric acid treatment on autogenous free graft coverage of localized recession. J Periodontol 1985;56:662–65.
23. Tolmie PN, Rubins RP, Buck GS, Vagianos V, Lanz JC. The predictability of root coverage by way of free gingival autografts and citric acid application: an evaluation by multiple clinicians. Int J Periodontics Restorative Dent 1991;11:261–71.
24. Grupe HE, Warren RF. Repair of gingival defects by a sliding flap operation. J Periodontol 1956;27:92–95.
25. Espinel MC, Caffesse RG. Lateral positioned pedicle sliding flap-revised technique in the treatment of localized gingival recessions. Int J Periodontics Restorative Dent 1981;1:43–51.
26. Guinard EA, Caffesse RG. Treatment of localized gingival recession. I. Lateral sliding flap. J Periodontol 1978;49:351–56.
27. Pennel BM, Higgason JD, Falder J, Towner J, King K, Fritz B. Oblique rotated flap. J Periodontol 1965;5: 36:305–8.
28. Smukler H. Laterally positioned mucoperiosteal pedicle grafts in the treatment of denuded roots. A clinical and statistical study. J Periodontol 1976;47: 590–95.
29. Caffesse RG, Alspach SR, Morrison EC, Burgett FG. Lateral sliding flaps with and without citric acid. Int J Periodontics Restorative Dent 1987;6:43–58.
30. Edel A. Clinical evaluation of free connective tissue grafts used to increase the width of keratinized gingiva. J Clin Periodontol 1974;1:185–89.
31. Raetzke PB. Covering localized areas of root exposure employing the envelope technique. J Periodontol 1985;56:397–402.
32. Langer B, Langer L. Subepithelial connective tissue graft technique for root coverage. J Periodontol 1985;56:715–20.
33. Nelson SW. The subepithelial connective tissue graft. A bilaminar reconstructive procedure for the coverage of denuded root surfaces. J Periodontol 1987;58:95–102.
34. Bruno J. Connective tissue graft technique assuring wide root coverage. Int J Periodont Rest Dent 1994;14: 127–37.
35. Reiser G M, Bruno J F. The sub epithelial connective tissue graft for achieving root coverage. Int J Periodont Rest Dent 1994;14:355–64.
36. Gottlow J, Nyman S, Karring T, Lindhe J. Treatment of localized gingival recessions with coronally displaced flaps and citric acid. An experimental study in the dog. J Clin Periodontol 1986;13:57–63.
37. Common J, McFall WT. The effect of citric acid on attachment of laterally repositioned flaps. J Periodontol 1983;54:9–19.
38. Pfeifer J, Heller R. Histologic evaluation of full and partial thickness lateral repositioned flaps. A pilot study. J Periodontol 1971;42:331–33.

39. Sugarman EF. A clinical and histological study of the attachment of grafted tissue to bone and teeth. J Periodontol 1969;40:381–87.

40. Tal H, Moses O, Zohar R, Meir H, Nemcovsky C. Root coverage of advanced gingival recession: A comparative study between acellular dermal matrix allograft and subepithelial connective tissue grafts. J Periodontl 2002;73:1405–11.

41. Callan DP, Silverstein LH. Use of acellular dermal matrix for increasing keratinized tissue around teeth and implants. Prac Periodontics Aesthet Dent 1998;10: 731–34.

42. Harris R. A comparative study of root coverage obtained with an acellular dermal matrix versus connective tissue grafts. Int J Periodontics Restorative Dent 2000;20:51–59.

43. Gottlow J, Nyman S, Lindhe J, Karring T, Wennstrom J. New attachment formation in the human periodontium by guided tissue regeneration. Case reports. J Clin Periodontol 1986;13:604–16.

44. Pini Prato GP, Tinti C, Vincenzi G, Magnani C, Cortellini P, Clauser C. Guided tissue regeneration versus mucogingival surgery in the treatment of human buccal gingival recession. J Periodontol 1992;63:919–28.

45. Pini Prato GP, Clauser C, Cortellini P. Resorbable membranes in the treatment of human buccal recession. A 9 case report. Int J Periodontics Restorative Dent 1995;15:259–68.

46. Roccuzzo M, Lungo M, Corrente G, Gandolfo S. Comparative study of a bioresorbable and a nonresorbable membrane in the treatment of human buccal gingival recessions. J Periodontol 1996;67: 7–14.

47. Tinti C, Vincenzi G, Cortellini P, Pini Prato G, Clauser C. Guided tissue regeneration in the treatment of human facial recession. A twelve-case report. J Periodontol 1992;63:54–60.

48. Tinti C, Vincenzi G. Expanded polytetrafluoroethylene titanium-reinforced membranes for regeneration of mucogingival recession defects. A 12-case report. J Periodontol 1994;65:1088–94.

49. Trombelli L, Tatakis DN, Scabbia A, Zimmerman GJ. Comparison of mucogingival changes following treatment with coronally positioned flap and guided tissue regeneration procedures. Int J Periodontics Restorative Dent 1997;17:448–55.

50. Trombelli L, Scabbia A, Tatakis DN, Checci L, Calura G. Resorbable barrier and envelope flap surgery in treatment of human gingival recession defects. Case reports. J Clin Periodontol 1998;25: 24–29.

51. Caffesse RG, Kon S, Castelli WA, Nasjleti CE. Revascularization following the lateral 51. sliding flap procedure. J Periodontol 1984;55:352–59.

52. Gottlow J, Nyman S, Karring T, Lindhe J. Treatment of localized gingival recessions with coronally displaced flaps and citric acid. An experimental study in the dog. J Clin Periodontol 1986;13:57–43.

53. Linghorne WJ, O'Connell DC. Studies in the regeneration and reattachment of supporting structures of the teeth. I. Soft tissue reattachment. J Dent Res 1950;29: 419–28.

54. Wilderman MN, Wentz FM. Repair of dentogingival defect with a pedicle flap. J Periodontol 1965;36: 218–31.

55. Woodyard SG, Snyder AJ, Henley G, O'Neal RB. A histometric evaluation of the effect of citric acid preparation upon healing of coronally positioned flaps in nonhuman primates. J Periodontol 1984;55: 203–12.

56. Common J, McFall WT. The effect of citric acid on attachment of laterally positioned flaps. J Periodontol 1983;54:9–18.

57. Cortellini P, Clauser C, Pini Prato G. Histologic assessment of new attachment following the treatment of a human buccal recession by means of a guided tissue regeneration procedure. J Periodontol 1993;64:387–91.

58. Pasquinelli KL. The histology of new attachment utilizing a thick autogenous soft tissue graft in an area of deep recession: A case report. Int J Periodontics Restorative Dent 1995;15:248–57

59. Pfeifer JA, Heller R. Histologic evaluation of full and partial thickness lateral repositioned flaps: a pilot study. J Periodontol 1971;42:331–33.

60. Sugarman EF. A clinical and histological study of the attachment of grafted tissue to bone and teeth. J Periodontol 1969;40:38–87.

61. Camargo P M, et al. The effectiveness of enamel matrix proteins used in combination with bovine porous bone mineral in the treatment of intrabony defects in humans. J Clin Periodontol 2001;28: 1016–22.

62. Cardaropoli G, Leonhardt A S. Enamel matrix proteins in the treatment of deep infrabony defects. J Periodontol 2002;73:501–4.

63. Cochran D L, et al. Periodontal regeneration with a combination of enamel matrix proteins and autogenous bone grafting. J Periodontol 2003;74: 1269–81.

64. Donos N, et al. Clinical evaluation of an enamel matrix derivative in the treatment of mandibular degree ii furcation involvement: A 36-month case series. Int J Periodontics Restorative Dent 2003;23: 507–12.

65. Francetti L, et al. Enamel matrix proteins in the treatment of intrabony defects—A prospective 24 months' clinical trial. J Clin Periodontol 2004;31: 52–59.

66. Froum S J, et al. The use of enamel matrix derivative in the treatment of periodontal osseous defects: A clinical decision tree based on biologic principles of regeneration. Int J Periodontics Restorative Dent 2001;21: 437–49.

67. Giannobile W, Somerman M. Growth and Amelogenin-like factors in periodontal wound healing. A systematic review. Ann Periodontol 2003;8: 193–204.

68. Heden G. A case report study of 72 consecutive emdogain-treated intrabony periodontal defects: Clinical and radiographic findings after 1 year. Int J Periodontics Restorative Dent 2000;20: 127–39.

69. Heijl L, et al. Enamel) in the treatment of intrabony periodontal(matrix derivative (EMDOGAIN defects. J Clin Periodontol 1997;24: 705–14.

70. Lekovic V, et al. Combination use of bovine porous bone mineral, enamel matrix proteins, and a bioabsorbable membrane in intrabony periodontal defects in humans. J Periodontol 2001;583–89.

71. Manor A. Periodontal regeneration with enamel matrix derivative—case reports. Int J Periodontics Restorative Dent 2000;20: 127–89.

72. Okuda K, et al. Enamel matrix derivative in the treatment of human intrabony periodontal osseous defects. J Periodontol 2000;71: 1821–28.

73. Parashis A, Tsiklakis K. Clinical and radiographic findings following application of enamel matrix derivative in treatment of intrabony defects. A series of case reports. J Clin Periodontol 2000;27: 705–13.

74. Rosen P S, Reynolds M A. A retrospective case series comparing the use of demineralized freeze-dried bone allograft and freeze-dried bone allograft combined with enamel matrix derivative for the treatment of advanced osseous lesions. J Periodontol 2002;73: 942–49.

75. Sculean A, et al. Treatment of intrabony defects with enamel matrix proteins and guided tissue regeneration. A prospective controlled clinical study. J Clin Periodontol 2001;28: 397–403.

76. Sculean A, et al. Treatment of intrabony defects with enamel matrix proteins or bioabsorbable membranes. A 4-year follow-up split-mouth study. J Periodontol 2001;72: 1695–701.

77. Sculean A, et al. Clinical evaluation of an enamel matrix protein derivative combined with a bioactive glass for the treatment of intrabony periodontal defects in humans. J Periodontol 2002;73: 401–8.

78. Sculean A, et al. Four-year results following treatment of intrabony periodontal defects with an enamel matrix protein derivative: a report of 46 cases. Int J Periodontics Restorative Dent 2003;23: 345–51.

79. Silvestri M, et al. Comparison of intrabony defects with enamel matrix derivative versus guided tissue regeneration with a nonresorbable membrane. A multicenter controlled clinical trial. J Clin Periodontol 2003;30: 386–93.

80. Tonetti M, et al. Enamel matrix proteins in the regenerative therapy of deep intrabony defects: A multicenter randomized controlled clinical trial. J Clin Periodontol 2002;29: 317–25.

81. Velasquez-Plata D, Scheyer E T, Mellonig J T. Clinical comparison of an enamel matrix derivative used alone or in combination with a bovine-derived xenograft for the treatment of periodontal osseous defects in humans. J Periodontol 2002;73: 433–40.

82. Windisch P, et al. Comparison of clinical, radiographic, and histometric measurements following treatment with guided tissue regeneration or enamel matrix proteins in human periodontal defects. J Periodontol 2002;73: 409–17.

83. Zucchelli G, et al. Enamel matrix protein and guided tissue regeneration with titanium-reinforced expanded polytetrafluoroethylene membranes in the treatment of infrabony defects: a comparative controlled clinical trial. J Periodontol 2002;73: 3–12.

84. Abbas F, et al. Surgical treatment of gingival recessions using Emdogain gel: Clinical procedure and case reports. Int J Periodontics Restorative Dent 2003;23: 607–13.

85. Berlucchi I, et al. Enamel matrix proteins (Emdogain) in combination with coronally advanced flap or subepithelial connective tissue graft in the treatment of shallow gingival recessions. Int J Periodontics Restorative Dent 2002;22: 3–13.

86. Carnio J, et al. histological evaluation of 4 cases of root coverage following a connective tissue graft combined with an enamel matrix derivative preparation. J Periodontol 2002;73: 1534–43

87. Hägewald S, et al. Comparative and coronally advanced flap technique in the treatment of(study of Emdogain human gingival recessions. A prospective controlled clinical study. J Clin Periodontol 2002;29: 35–41.

88. McGuire M K, Nunn M. Evaluation of human recession defects treated with coronally advanced flaps and either enamel matrix derivative or connective tissue. Part I: Comparison of clinical parameters. J Periodontol 2003;74: 1110–25.

89. Modica F, et al. Coronally advanced flap for the treatment of buccal gingival recessions with and without enamel matrix derivative. A split-mouth study. J Periodontol 2000;71: 1693–98.

90. Siervo S, Coraini C. Muco-gingival and regenerative therapy with amelogenins. Dental Cadmus 1998;20: 37–42.

91. Hammarström L, Heijl L, Gestrelius S. Periodontal regeneration in a buccal dehiscence model in monkeys after application of enamel matrix proteins. J Clin Periodontol 1997;24: 669–77.

92. McGuire M K, Cochran D L. Evaluation of human recession defects treated with coronally advanced flaps and either enamel matrix derivative or connective tissue. Part 2: Histological evaluation. J Periodontol 2003;74: 1126–35.

93. Mellonig J. Enamel matrix derivative for periodontal reconstructive surgery: technique and clinical and histologic case report. Int J Periodontics Restorative Dent 1999;19: 9–19.

94. Parodi R, et al. Use of Emdogain in the treatment of deep intrabony defects: 12-month clinical results. Histologic and radiographic evaluation. Int J Periodontics Restorative Dent 2000;20: 585–95.

95. Rasperini G, et al. Clinical and histologic evaluation of human gingival recession treated with a subepithelial connective tissue graft and enamel matrix derivative (Emdogain): A case report. Int J Periodontics Restorative Dent 2000;20: 269–74.

96. Sculean A, et al. Healing of recession-type defects following treatment with enamel matrix proteins or guided tissue regeneration. A pilot study in monkeys. Journal de Parodontologie & D'impantologie Orale 2000;19 (1);19–31.

97. Yukna R A, Mellonig J. Histological evaluation of periodontal healing in humans following regenerative therapy with enamel matrix derivative. A 10-case series. J Periodontol 2000;71: 752–59

98. Marx RE, Carlson ER, Eichstaedt RM, Schimmele SR,Strauss JE, Geuseffe KR. Platelet-rich plasma: Growth factors enhancement for bone grafts. Oral Surg Oral Med Oral Pathol Oral Radiol Endodon. 1998;85:63–46.

99. Rai B, Teoh SH, Ho KH. An in vitro evaluation of PCL-TCP composites as delivery systems for platelet rich plasma. J Control Rel. 2005;107:330–42.

100. Yamada Y, Ueda M, Hibi H, Baba S. A novel approach to periodontal tissue regeneration with mesenchymal stem cells and platelet-rich plasma using technology: A clinical case report. Int J Periodontics Restorative Dent 2006;26:363–69.

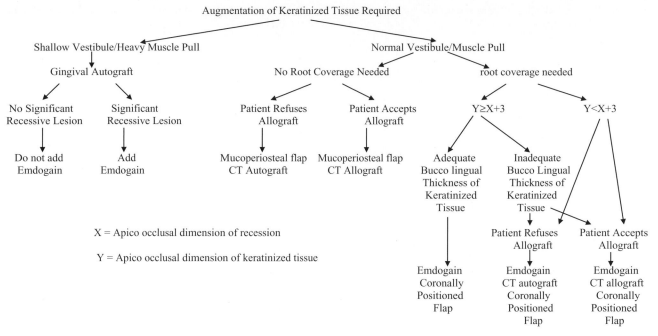

Flow chart 4.1 Treating mucogingival problems.

Chapter 5
Restoration of the Periodontally Treated Tooth

Frederick Hains

Conservation of tooth structure while achieving a return to form and function with a lasting prosthetic restorative procedure are the goals of the restorative dentist. The approach taken with direct or indirect restorative procedures is aimed at the recapture of oral health and long-term stability, through the use of materials that will replace missing or damaged tooth structure without violation of biological tenets or compromise of mechanical principles.

Because emphasis is placed on conservation in the modern concepts of tooth preparation, many of the G. V. Black principles of cavity preparation have been put aside (1). Improvements in dental materials and evidence-based procedures have shown minimally invasive treatments to be meritorious. It is a well-accepted concept that naturally occurring tooth structure is superior to its artificial substitutes. Therefore, tooth preparation decisions are made that tend to preserve tooth structure, protect vital pulpal structures, avoid violation of the periodontium, and reestablish healthy contacts with the neighboring teeth.

The concepts of retention and resistance form must be emphasized while mastering various tooth preparation designs for partial and full-coverage restorations, as well as the unique preparation requirements for ceramics and CAD/CAM materials.

A partial-coverage approach is employed where possible, and the taper of the preparation is kept to a minimal convergence angle. Tooth reduction follows the external anatomy of the tooth, and should be uniform and appropriate for the materials chosen to replace the prepared tooth structure. Aesthetic demands must be taken into account. Overreduction, whether occlusally or axially, will jeopardize the integrity and health of the pulpal tissues and will require sophisticated laboratory skills in the fabrication of the resulting prosthesis. Optimal tooth reduction maximizes aesthetic results and culminates in a durable, long-lasting restoration. This objective is achieved by the proper tooth preparation and margin design.

An acceptable restorative margin would have a margin design that results in the smallest cement gap or space possible, that achieves the desired aesthetics for the situation, and that falls into an area free of recurrent disease that is easy to maintain. An ideal margin demonstrates the following characteristics:

- It is easy to prepare.
- It is easy to see in the impression and on the prepared tooth.
- The prepared margin results in a dies that can be easily read.
- The preparation depth is sufficient to result in adequate metal thickness or porcelain bulk to avoid distortion and to achieve aesthetics appropriate for the given situation.

The three major preparation geometries are: the feather, the chamfer, and the shoulder. These preparation designs are distinguished by their unique marginal geometries (Figs. 5.1–5.4).

The Feather

The feather margin preparation design conserves the most tooth structure of all preparation designs. Margin preparation is made with a tapered bur. Axial reduction is minimal, as the goal of the

Periodontal Restorative Interrelationships: Ensuring Clinical Success, First Edition. Edited by Paul A. Fugazzotto.
© 2011 by John Wiley & Sons, Inc. Published 2011 by John Wiley & Sons, Inc.

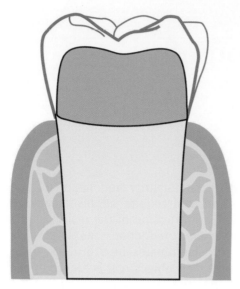

Fig. 5.1 A diagrammatic representation of a feather-edge margin.

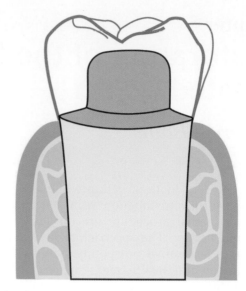

Fig. 5.3 A diagrammatic representation of a shoulder margin.

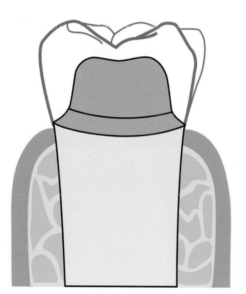

Fig. 5.2 A diagrammatic representation of chamfer margin.

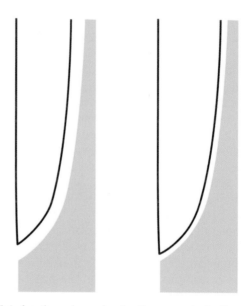

Fig. 5.4 Another view of a feather margin in the seating process.

feather edge margin preparation is conservative removal of tooth structure and maximization of the retentive nature of the preparation through the use of a minimal taper. This margin preparation is difficult to accomplish because it is difficult to see. The distinct boundary between the prepared tooth structure and the unprepared tooth structure can seem obscure.

The feather edge margin is indicated in those situations where the need for tooth structure conservation and a retentive preparation are crucial. A situation where the structure of a tooth to be restored is short incisogingivally will benefit from this style of preparation. The minimal taper of the design adds retentive form to the preparation. The feather edge margin design is also employed when the teeth being prepared are long and narrow (Figs. 5.5–5.8). The more aggressive margin preparations to be discussed, with the exception of the light chamfer, are contra-indicated

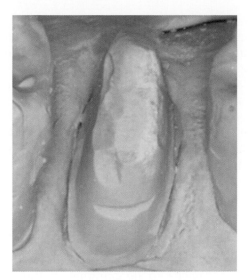

Fig. 5.5 A view of the model after impression is poured in stone.

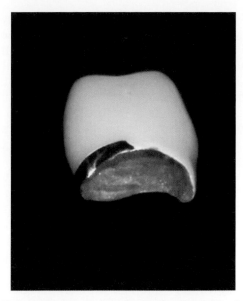

Fig. 5.7 A view of the crown for the prepared tooth.

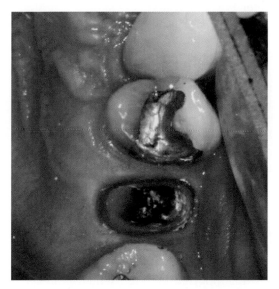

Fig. 5.6 A tooth preparation with a feather-edge margin has been carried out. Note the long parallel preparation, which is necessary for retention.

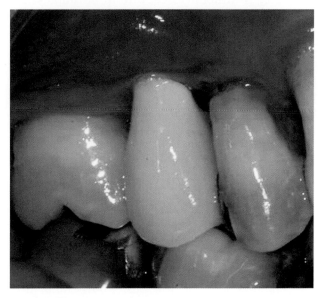

Fig. 5.8 The crown is delivered.

in such situations as they require too great a degree of tooth structure removal at the cervical aspect of the tooth and would compromise the integrity of the pulpal tissue. This preparation design is employed in areas of severe recession, when the preparation margin must be placed on root structure. For obvious reasons, the preparation needs to be minimal and be placed supragingivally. The profile of the finished restoration must be

flat, and emergence from the gingival to the incisal aspects of the crown must be devoid of plaque trapping contours. This area is sensitive to additional attachment loss and must be protected during the impression making process by avoiding invasions of the sulcus with retraction media. The restoration should finish with a polished margin that has minimal plaque retentive properties.

The feather edge preparation is employed in areas where the furcation has been exposed, or where there has been excessive recession and the root surface has to be prepared. The minimal axial tooth reduction of the feather edge design both prevents the development of tooth preparation undercuts and avoids overpreparation of thin residual tooth structure. Such margins are placed supragingivally so as to be more easily examined and managed.

While the feather edge margin design has the advantages of being minimally invasive and improving the retention and resistance form of a tooth preparation, the difficulties one experienced in the laboratory phase of restoration makes this a margin preparation to be employed only in specific circumstances.

The feather edge is a difficult design for the laboratory to work with in the fabrication of a restoration. The tooth preparation, with a minimal distinction between prepared and unprepared tooth structure, is difficult to capture in an impression. This visual obscurity translates to the dies, where the margin is more difficult to see. If the margin is misread and is thought to extend more apically than it does, there is the potential for the restoration to fail to seat on the tooth. Conversely, if the margin is read as short of the actual finish line, the resulting restoration will seal the prepared area just short of the true finish line, which can be acceptable.

The laboratory will also be challenged in the fabrication of a restoration using the lost wax method, as the wax at the marginal area is thin and easily broken or distorted.

The Chamfer

The chamfer may be the best known and most popular preparation design in clinical practice, as it is easy to place and can be readily identified on the tooth and in the impression. The resulting die is easy to read. There is a distinct boundary between prepared and unprepared tooth structure, which may be predictably captured in a wax pattern. The chamfer preparation has sufficient depth to ensure that the resultant wax pattern and castings are stable and can be handled without distortion.

The internal anatomy of the chamfer preparation is obtained with a round-ended bur, as rounded internal angles are the preferred design. The rounded internal angle design has the favorable attribute of distributing forces rather than concentrating them, an attribute that is important when porcelain is added to the framework for a porcelain metal restoration. The inclined nature of the semi-circular design ensures positive seating of the restoration and a closed marginal gap. The chamfer preparation design is aesthetic when placed in healthy periodontal environments, 0.5 mm into the sulcus of anterior teeth

The chamfer has a versatility not seen in any of the other preparation designs. Because the preparation mirrors a round-ended bur, the diameter of the bur used will dictate the axial depth of the preparation. Therefore, in the instance where the preparation needs to be minimal, a thin round-ended diamond bur is selected. In a situation where a deeper axial preparation is required to allow maximum thickness of porcelain, a larger diameter bur is selected.

However, a weakness of the chamfer preparation is also contained in the round-ended bur that creates the preparation. The ideal margin design requires a preparation that is actually less than the diameter of the bur, which can be technically difficult for the operator to accomplish. If the depth of the preparation penetrates beyond the diameter of the bur, a reverse curve is created in the marginal area, resulting in a tooth "lip," which will hamper the fabrication of a stable die margin or wax pattern, and will create a casting that will not seat completely. The occurrence of this enamel lip is greatest when axial penetration increases. Therefore, the smallest error will have the most profound affect (Fig. 5.9).

In such a situation, the margin edge demonstrates unsupported enamel, which is not a stable situation and cannot be accurately reproduced by the laboratory. The use of a bevel eliminates this problem and improves the fit of the restoration. The subcategory of beveled margins is of great advantage with the heavy chamfered margin design.

The Shoulder

The shoulder preparation is performed with a tapered, flat-ended bur, resulting in an axial wall that tapers in an occlusal direction from a flat gingival cervical floor. The preparation is easy to

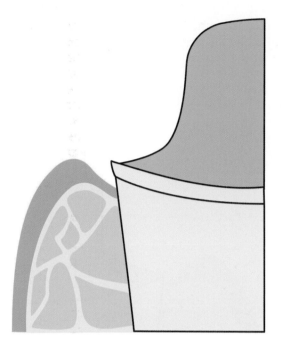

Fig. 5.9 An example of overpreparation resulting in a reverse curve or lip.

distinguish, as there is a distinct boundary between prepared and unprepared tooth structure. The shoulder preparation has sufficient depth to ensure that the resulting wax pattern and castings are stable and can be easily handled without distortion.

The shoulder preparation needs to be placed at or slightly coronal to the marginal gingiva in order to achieve clarity of the finish line. The blunt cervical margin, when prepared to an adequate axial depth, can be restored in metal, ceramometal, or porcelain. The marginal geometry of the shoulder design makes it accepting of all porcelain margins, with the aesthetic advantage of allowing placement of a bulk of porcelain. Increased strength and designed optical properties are attained through such placement of bulk material at the cervical aspect of the tooth. This fact is crucial, as the cervical aspect of a prepared tooth is an area where opaque show through may betray an otherwise aesthetic restoration as being inadequately reduced.

The draw back to the shoulder design is that it is an aggressive and difficult preparation to execute. The marginal finish must be smooth and free of areas of unsupported enamel. When preparing a tooth, marginal placement angulates from the buccal in an occlusal direction through the interdental spaces, and terminates on the lingual aspect of the tooth. Creating a continuously flat surface in a 360-degree tooth-bound space requires a certain level of skill.

Another drawback to the shoulder design is the difficulty in capturing it in an impression. In circumstances where there is little space between the marginal tissue and the finished margin, marginal material tears and inaccuracies within the impression may occur. The resultant dies will reflect these inaccuracies. Because there is a flush right-angle fit of restorative material to tooth surface, any distortions will result in an open margin or a failure of the restoration to seal.

Considering the context of the distortions inherent in impression materials, die fabrication materials, and restorative materials, this concern is a considerable impediment to overcome (Fig. 5.10).

To overcome these shortcomings and improve preparation marginal design, a subcategory has evolved that incorporates the use of a beveled margin. Such a bevel has great application with the heavy shoulder margin design.

BEVELED MARGINS AS A SUBCATEGORY

Marginal areas that will be required to support porcelain need to have a design that permits the laboratory to fabricate a substructure with sufficient strength to prevent distortion in the fabrication of the restoration, flexure at delivery of the restoration, and destabilization of the porcelain at the porcelain metal interface. The use of the bevel as a subcategory in the shoulder or heavy chamfer design combines the positive aspects of these two major preparation design categories, resulting in

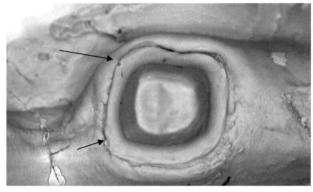

Fig. 5.10 A view of the die of a shoulder preparation without a bevel. Note the errors that are present.

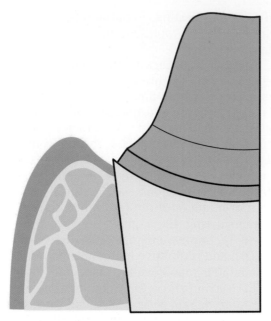

Fig. 5.11 A diagrammatic representation of a heavy chamfer with a bevel.

aesthetics, increased retention, and ease of impressioning (Fig. 5.11).

All porcelain margins represent another possible solution to this problem. However, to ensure an adequate and stable margin, a preparation that provides for adequate thickness of porcelain at the margin also creates a marginal gap, which represents an inherent compromise.

The best solution to aesthetic margin placement is the use of metal at the tooth restoration interface, due to the accuracy of the casting and design of the metal at the margin to support the porcelain. The margin design of choice has traditionally been a heavy chamfer, which provides for the required thickness of material at the margin for stability of the restoration's margin, and porcelain placement with an improved tooth restoration gap over the all-porcelain margin. This design also has a rounded axial gingival contour, which is more favorable to the placement and support of porcelain. Due to the semicircular nature of the margin design, the fit is optimized and marginal gap is minimized by concept of inclined planes. This concept states that surfaces that meet on inclined planes will be closed at some point along that incline.

The shoulder design will allow for adequate marginal dimensions to place metal and porcelain,

or all porcelain, margins. However, because the final marginal design is at right angles to the long axis of the tooth, the fit of such a margin is often less accurate than desired, resulting in an unacceptable margin gap (Figs. 5.12, 5.13).

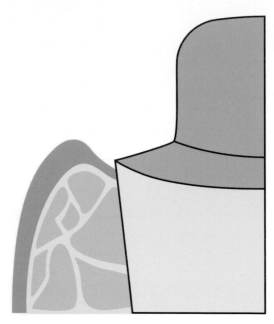

Fig. 5.12 A diagrammatic representation of a shoulder preparation.

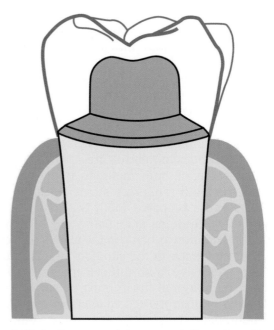

Fig. 5.13 A diagrammatic representation of a shoulder preparation with a bevel preparation.

To overcome this drawback of the shoulder design, and improve the fit of the restoration, a bevel is placed 0.5 mm into the sulcus. The aesthetics of the porcelain at the margin, coupled with the fit of a beveled margin hidden in the sulcus, has proven to be a successful solution to this quandary.

Such a bevel has also been applied to the heavy chamfer margin design taking advantage of the curved internal angles of the preparation, which favor the placement and support of porcelain, and the aesthetics achieved by hiding the margin in the sulcus. The use of a bevel adds to the retentive nature of the preparation. In areas where dislodging stresses require compensatory resistance to dislodgment, the use of a bevel adds extra resistance form.

These two designs that employ a bevel offer the added advantage of opening the sulcus for the placement of impression materials. When making an impression in the case of a heavy chamfer or shoulder preparation, the gap between the sulcus and the prepared margin is narrow. Even when the soft tissues are retracted, the tissues will rebound, resulting in a thin deposit of impression material at that critical junction. The resultant impression may tear at the tooth margin gingival interface because this area could not receive sufficient impression material bulk. A bevel opens this environment and allows the sulcus to receive impression material in sufficient quantity to avoid tearing and to provide more accurate detail (Figs. 5.14, 5.15).

A literature review conducted in 2001 "suggested that margin design selection should be based on the type of crown, applicable aesthetic requirements, ease of formation and operator's experience. The expectation of enhanced fit based on a particular marginal geometry was not validated" (2).

Knowledge of how to apply various marginal geometries, and an understanding of the advantages and limitations of each approach, affords the clinician the freedom to select marginal designs and utilize them where they offer the greatest advantage and will provide the desired outcome. It is critically important to have the flexibility of using various margin designs in the preparation of a tooth, as a particular tooth may require several different marginal geometries to achieve an optimal result. An example is the maxillary first premolar. The anatomy of this tooth does not lend itself to

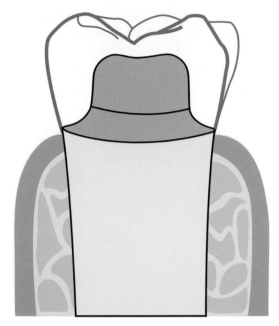

Fig. 5.14 A diagrammatic representation of a crown seated on an unbeveled heavy chamfer preparation.

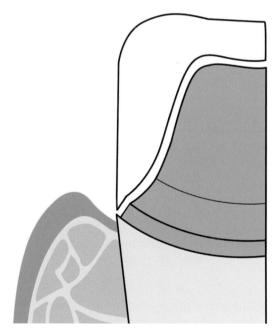

Fig. 5.15 A diagrammatic representation of a crown seating on a beveled preparation.

a 360-degree aggressive, aesthetic preparation, be it a shoulder or a heavy chamfer. There may be sufficient tooth structure to permit a shoulder or heavy chamfer preparation on the facial aspect of the tooth. However, the mesial root groove/furcation, and the resultant thin tooth structure in this area, require a less aggressive preparation to fulfill the principles of conservation of tooth structure and protection of the pulpal tissues. Additionally, it is unnecessary to aggressively prepare the distal, proximal, or lingual areas of the maxillary first premolar, as they are often not in the aesthetic zone and can therefore be prepared with a much gentler and less aggressive marginal geometry. By utilizing knowledge of the various marginal geometries, and coupling that knowledge with the necessary skills to execute the various marginal designs, the clinician might select the use of a heavy chamfer for the mesiobuccal aspect of the maxillary first premolar, taper to a chamfer preparation that would be carried distally into the distal interproximal space and on to the lingual tooth structure, and culminate in a feather preparation through the mesial interproximal area and the furcation area where the tooth structure is thin in an axial direction. The margin would then terminate at the buccal inset of the heavy buccal chamfer.

The heavy chamfer will permit optimal aesthetics by providing adequate tooth reduction in an area that has the greatest visual impact, and affording the dental laboratory the opportunity to fabricate an aesthetic restoration with the proper ceramic dimensions. The use of a chamfer at the distal, interproximal, and lingual surfaces of the tooth takes advantage of a marginal design that is less invasive and preserves tooth structure, while allowing for aesthetics where the demand is not as great as the mesiobuccal aspect of the tooth. Finally, the most demanding anatomical area of the tooth can be prepared with a marginal geometry that avoids undercuts, is minimally invasive, allows preparation into the furcation, avoids leaving tooth lips, and provides for a flat, healthier emergence profile.

Consideration of margin designs is not complete without a discussion of all ceramic restorations. The early all-ceramic restorations presented with significant shortcomings, as they required exacting marginal geometry and accurate impressions to capture that preparation. The marginal geometry was either a shoulder or heavy chamfer preparation. The ceramic material gathered its

strength from bulk and avoidance of sharp internal angles, which tended to concentrate stresses within the ceramic material. Failure to adhere to the preparation guidelines for a ceramic restoration led to fracture of the restoration. The risk for failure limited the use of ceramic restoration to the anterior zone, where the stresses of occlusion were less and the demands of the preparation were easier to accomplish. The reward was generally a more aesthetically pleasing restoration. The presence of a large margin gap required the use of cements that were aesthetic, non–water soluble, strong, and did not expand over time. Resin cements were championed as an answer to the marginal weakness of the all-ceramic restoration.

Newer ceramics are stronger. In addition, the use of milling or pressing technologies with ceramic materials has improved the accuracy of the fit, lowered the marginal gap size, and reduced the need for aggressive tooth preparation. Fortified ceramics such as zirconium and lava have the strength of metal and can be used in areas where preparations are minimal. The recommended marginal reduction is now in the range of 1.25 mm, which represents a 60% less aggressive preparation than the 2 mm or better of tooth reduction required for ceramometal restorations. Load-bearing areas require 1.50 mm to 2.00 mm of reduction for a ceramic crown, which is the same requirement called for with ceramometal restorations.

Periodontal Ramifications and Prosthetic Adaptations

Prosthetic preparation of tooth structure in a healthy environment with no history of disease requires knowledge of the restorative materials chosen, as well as the marginal geometry necessary to achieve the restorative endpoint. Unfortunately, this is frequently not the environment the clinician faces. Most often the area in need of prosthetic therapy demonstrates loss of attachment apparatus, and the clinician is confronted with the tooth root anatomy, in addition to the coronal tooth structure. The furcations of multirooted teeth introduce a complexity to tooth preparation that is all too often missed or disregarded. The naturally occurring undercut, or "furcation roof" of a multirooted tooth that has suffered attachment loss and exposure of the furcation must be considered and treated in the preparation of these teeth.

For a discussion of furcation classifications, see Chapter 3.

A molar with multiple roots, around which attachment and bone loss have not occurred, permits a straightforward approach to the preparation of the tooth. Reduction that is uniform, appropriate, and anatomically directed, with marginal geometry suitable for the projected restorative goal, is indicated. However, when the milieu requires a preparation that includes the area below the cementoenamel junction (CEJ) and involves the root system, the restorative dentist must have a keen understanding of the anatomy of the tooth and the restorative options available to fit the particular circumstances.

When the furcation in question is periodontally involved, a restorative form must be employed in these instances, which will be conducive to the health of the area and will not trap plaque or impede a patient's ability to maintain the area.

The ability to anticipate the restorative complexities that may be encountered is grounded in an understanding of molar root anatomy. The general configuration of the maxillary molar root system includes a palatal root, which is wide buccolingually and mesiodistally and which diverges palatally from the crown. The mesiobuccal and distobuccal roots are biconcave and have a distal curvature of varying degree towards the distal. Second and third maxillary molars root configurations are more likely to have fused roots than first molars. The location of the distal furcation is more apical than that of the mesial furcation. Treatment of a maxillary molar with furcation involvement is realistic and predictable, provided that the prepared tooth configuration is in an easily cleansable area and is manageable for the patient. Such a goal that may mandate removal of a root has been discussed in Chapter 3.

The mandibular molar generally is found with two roots, the mesial root and the distal root. The mesial root has a flattened appearance buccolingually with a concave proximal surface on each side of the root. This root generally curves distally. The distal root is more robust than the mesial root, being wider buccolingually, and usually has a proximal concavity only on the mesial aspect of the root (Fig. 5.16).

The proximal concavities found on the mesial and distal roots create an osseous chamber in the area where the roots divide from the crown. This area is wider mesiodistally than either the lingual

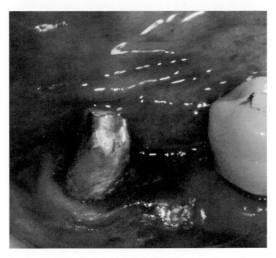

Fig. 5.16 A clinical view of the distal root of tooth number 19.

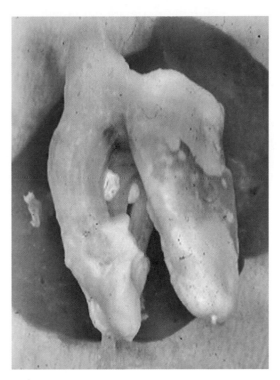

Fig. 5.17 A view of the interradicular anatomy of an extracted molar.

or buccal furcation openings and poses a potential restorative problem when it is exposed following attachment loss. If this area is left intact, it cannot be restored predictably. In addition, achieving an acceptable flat emergence profile that is not plaque retentive and is cleansable is difficult or impossible in this scenario, because of the anatomy of the interradicular space (Figs. 5.17, 5.19, 5.20).

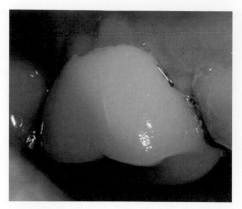

Fig. 5.18 An all-porcelain crown has been inserted with a supragingival margin.

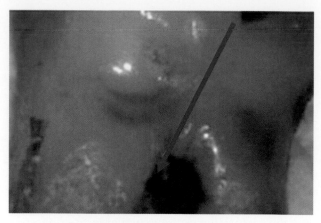

Fig. 5.19 A view of a furcation.

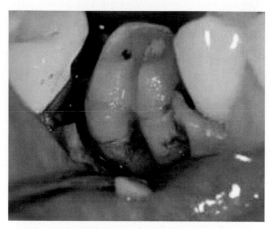

Fig. 5.20 Tooth preparation has been accomplished at the furcation area.

A maxillary or mandibular molar with a Class I furcation will require a marginal crown preparation that includes the furcation, or that is far enough coronal to the furcation as to not be involved in its anatomy. Fig. 5.18 demonstrates an all-ceramic crown placed coronal to the buccal furcation.

As the root trunk of a tooth emerges from the coronal structure of the molar, at the point of definition of the root into a mesial and distal root system for mandibular molars, or a mesial buccal, distal buccal, and palatal root system for maxillary molars, there is an anatomical concavity that develops and increases in an apical direction until there is separation of the individual roots. As a result, the natural protective curvatures of the tooth are no longer effective at directing food away from the cervical areas of the tooth once recession has exposed the root trunk area of the molar. Additionally, the naturally occurring undercut of the root trunk area is plaque retentive. Therefore, the prosthetic crown contours must be adapted to reestablish a form that will provide protection from insult and minimize plaque retention. A treated Class I furcation involvement is managed by increasing the axial-coronal preparation in the area coronal to the reshaped furcation region, permitting the fabrication of a crown with a flat emergence profile coronally to ensure that there is no undercut to trap food or plaque (Figs. 5.19–5.21).

As discussed in Chapter 3, molars are not the only teeth with furcations or root anatomies that must be taken into consideration when full-coverage restoration is anticipated.

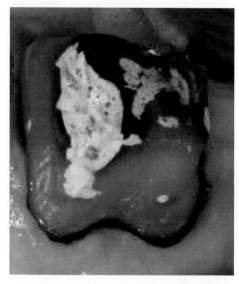

Fig. 5.21 A view of the marginal preparation in the area of the furcation.

When restoring multirooted bicuspids, the principles remain the same. The objective is to create a sealed marginal area and a crown profile that are conducive to maintenance and lack plaque retentive areas.

When faced with deeper furcation involvements, the restorative dentist, periodontist, and endodontist may elect to reconfigure the anatomy of the tooth by removal of a root, to eliminate the furcation. Following maxillary molar root resection, the marginal preparation must be minimal, as it occurs on root structure, and the tooth root dimensions will not allow aggressive preparations. The area where the root was removed must be prepared in a fashion that allows for a flat emergence profile and manageable surfaces that can be kept plaque free (Figs. 5.22–5.24).

Following mandibular molar root resection, the preparation of the remaining root structure must utilize a preparation geometry that minimizes the depth of the margin placement and eliminates root concavities to create flat emergence profiles, which are easy to maintain. In such a situation, a feather margin preparation is indicated.

Preparation design is influenced by the unique anatomical features of each tooth type, the extensive periodontal therapy that has been performed, and the planned restoration (Tables 5.1–5.6).

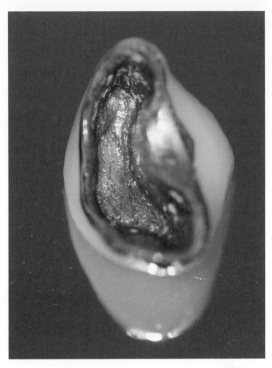

Fig. 5.23 A view of the underside of the casting demonstrates the adaptation of the marginal crown form to the prepared tooth morphology.

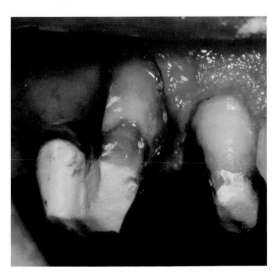

Fig. 5.22 The maxillary right first molar has undergone a distal buccal root amputation with appropriate periodontal therapy and tooth preparation. In this case, the tooth was to be crowned after resection therapy.

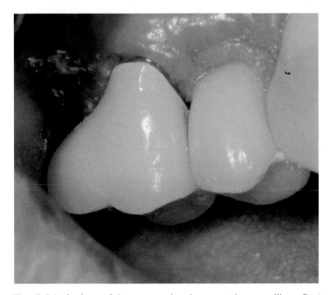

Fig. 5.24 A view of the crown in place on the maxillary first molar. Note the flat emergence profile of the restoration as it exits the gingiva, thus enhancing patient plaque control efforts.

Table 5.1. Preparation options for maxillary anterior teeth.

Tissue profile	Preparation design	Restoration of choice
Healthy, thick biotype	Chamfer or shoulder	All-ceramic restoration PFM an alternative, with a beveled buccal margin hidden in the sulcus, or a buccal butt porcelain finish
Healthy, thin biotype	Buccal heavy chamfer margin placed at the gingival margin Chamfer through the interproximal and on the lingual surfaces	All ceramic restoration PFM an alternative with porcelain butt buccal margin If a PFM is required, a heavy chamfer is the margin of choice on the buccal and chamfer margin through the interproximal and onto the lingual surface.
Recession and attachment loss; long tooth; open embrasures	Buccal chamfer margin placed at the gingival margin Chamfer through the interproximal and on the lingual surfaces May be necessary to use a light chamfer to avoid overpreparation at the cervical and at undercuts in the long axis of the tooth Margin placed at the gingival margin	PFM with buccal porcelain coverage Polished collars at the margin interproximally and lingually

Table 5.2. Preparation options for maxillary premolar teeth.

Tissue profile	Preparation design	Restoration of choice
Healthy, thick biotype	Chamfer or shoulder	All-ceramic restoration PFM an alternative, with a beveled buccal margin hidden in the sulculus
Healthy, thin biotype	Buccal heavy chamfer margin placed at the gingival margin Chamfer through the interproximal and on the lingual surfaces Mesiobuccal aspect prepared more aggressively, less so distally and interproximally	All-ceramic restoration PFM an alternative, with porcelain butt buccal margin If a PFM is required, heavy chamfer is the margin of choice on the mesiobuccal, and a chamfer margin through the distal, interproximal, and the lingual.
Recession and attachment loss; long tooth; open embrasures	Chamfer preparation on the mesial buccal Light chamfer through the distal interproximal Feather or light chamfer in the mesial furcation area, being sure to keep a flat emergence profile in the mesial furcation area Finish line would be supragingival Cervical depth of the prepared tooth minimal to protect pulpal health and avoid undercuts	PFM restoration Metal support is required in areas where the axial reduction is minimal.

Table 5.3. Preparation options for maxillary molar teeth.

Tissue profile	Preparation design	Restoration of choice
Healthy, thick biotype	Chamfer or shoulder, with modified mesiobuccal reduction to maximize aesthetics	Reinforced ceramic restoration if reduction and margin placement allow PFM alternative, with beveled buccal margin hidden in the sulcus
Healthy, thin biotype	Buccal heavy chamfer placed at the gingival margin Chamfer through the interproximal and on the lingual surfaces Mesiobuccal aspect is prepared more aggressively, less so moving distal and interproximal.	Reinforced ceramic restoration with supragingival finish same requirements as above PFM alternative, with porcelain butt buccal margin If a PFM is required, heavy chamfer margin on the mesiobuccal, and chamfer margin through the mesial and distal interproximal areas and on the lingual
Recession and attachment loss; long tooth; open embrasures	Chamfer preparation on the mesial buccal Light chamfer through the mesial and distal interproximal areas Feather or light chamfer in the interproximal areas Flat emergence profile in the furcation areas Feather margin will be necessary should the recession be extreme. Finish line supragingival Cervical depth of the prepared tooth minimal to protect pulpal health and avoid undercuts	PFM restoration Metal support required in thin areas where the axial reduction must be minimal

Table 5.4. Preparation options for mandibular anterior teeth.

Tissue profile	Preparation design	Restoration of choice
Healthy, thick biotype	Difficult tooth to prepare Thin tooth structure requires a minimal chamfer aesthetic preparation	Reinforced ceramic restoration PFM an alternative, with a beveled buccal margin hidden in the sulcus
Healthy, thin biotype	Buccal heavy chamfer margin placed at the gingival margin Light chamfer through the interproximal and on the lingual surfaces	Reinforced ceramic restoration only if the margin depth can be uniform PFM an alternative, with porcelain butt buccal margin If PFM is required, heavy chamfer is the margin of choice on the buccal and light chamfer or feather margin through the interproximal and on the lingual.
Recession and attachment loss; long tooth; open embrasures	Buccal chamfer margin placed at the gingival margin Chamfer through the interproximal and on the lingual May be necessary to use a light chamfer to avoid overpreparation at the cervical area and at undercuts in the long axis of the tooth Margin placed at the gingival margin	PFM with buccal porcelain coverage Minimal metal collar Polished collars at the margins interproximally and lingually Aesthetics give way to preservation of tooth structure.

Table 5.5. Preparation options for mandibular premolar teeth.

Tissue profile	Preparation design	Restoration of choice
Healthy, thick biotype	Chamfer or shoulder	All-ceramic restoration PFM an alternative, with a beveled buccal margin hidden in the sulcus
Healthy, thin biotype	Buccal heavy chamfer margin at the gingival margin Chamfer through the interproximal and on the lingual Mesial bucco is prepared more aggressively, less so distally and interproximally.	All ceramic restoration PFM an alternative, with porcelain butt buccal margin If a PFM is required, heavy chamfer is the margin of choice on the mesiobuccal, and chamfer margin through the distal and interproximal and on the lingual.
Recession and attachment loss; long tooth; open embrasures	Chamfer preparation on the mesiobuccal Light chamfer in the mesial interproximal area Flat emergence profile in the mesial furcation area	PFM restoration Metal support is required in thin areas where axial reduction must be minimal.

Table 5.6. Preparation options for mandibular premolar teeth.

Tissue profile	Preparation design	Restoration of choice
Healthy, thick biotype	Chamfer or shoulder Modified mesial buccal reduction to maximize aesthetics	All-ceramic restoration, if reduction and margin placement allows PFM an alternative, with a beveled buccal margin hidden in the sulcus
Healthy, thin biotype	Buccal heavy chamfer placed at the gingival margin Chamfer through the interproximal and on the lingual Mesiobuccal aspect is prepared more aggressively, less so distally and interproximally.	All-ceramic restoration with a supragingival finish, same requirement as above PFM an alternative, with porcelain butt buccal margin If a PFM is required, heavy chamfer is the margin of choice on the mesiobuccal, and the chamfer margin through to the distal and both interproximal areas and the lingual.
Recession and attachment loss; long tooth; open embrasures	Chamfer preparation on the mesiobuccal Light chamfer through the distal interproximal Feather or light chamfer in the mesial interproximal area Flat emergence profile in the mesial and buccal furcation areas Feather margin will be necessary if recession is extreme. Finish is supragingival. Cervical depth of the prepared tooth minimal to protect pulpal health and avoid undercuts Flat emergence profile to avoid plaque retention	PFM restoration Metal support is required in the thin areas where the axial reduction must be minimal.

Impressions

IMPRESSION MAKING

One of the many important steps in the production of an indirect restoration is the making of an impression of the tooth preparations and reproducing this preparation effort into a medium that can be used by the dental laboratory for the fabrication of the final restoration. An accurate, flexible flowable medium is utilized, which will capture the tooth preparations and adjacent dental and soft-tissue structures, permitting the fabrication of a model that will mimic the intraoral condition and allow the dental laboratory to fabricate an accurate restoration. While understanding the properties of the materials employed in making an impression may seem obvious, there are many options to assess. Factors that need to be considered in the making of an accurate impression are:

1. Selection of the tray or conveyance that will carry the impression material to the site to be impressed.
2. Selection of the appropriate elastomeric materials to be used in the impression-making process.
3. Manipulation of the soft tissues to produce an accurate replica of the submarginal environment. The detail obtained from this part of the impression provides critical tooth contour, emergence profile, gingival tissue position, and margin geometry information.
4. Delivery of the impression materials to the site in a manner aimed at achieving optimal results.

Impression material needs to be transported to the patient in a vessel that will permit ease of insertion into the mouth and will be of sufficient strength to ensure that no deformation occurs during placement or removal from the mouth. The conveyance must afford the impression material sufficient and uniform room to capture the dental structures accurately and in their entirety. The use of custom trays is advocated, as they fit the specific anatomy of the patient. When made correctly, custom trays provide the proper stops to prevent overseating of the tray and, with the usage of a measured spacer, proper volume of material to be placed around the prepared and unprepared teeth, so as to minimize distortions due to material excesses and deficiencies (Table 5.7).

Table 5.7. Impression tray selection.

Tray type	Advantage	Disadvantage	Indication	Contraindications
Custom	Improved accuracy due to material control and custom fit	Fabrication time and anticipation of the need for the tray	All areas of the mouth	None
Stock plastic	Inexpensive No need to preplan	Flexible Unstable in the mouth Subject to distortion Lack of uniformity of impression material within the tray	Preliminary impressions	Edentulous areas that are not tooth boarded Second molar preparations
Quadrant plastic	Inexpensive No need to preplan	Flexible Unstable in the mouth Subject to distortion Lack of uniformity of impression material within the tray Mounting errors due to lack of tooth contacts	None	All prosthetic impression situations
Metal	Stable material No need to preplan	Lack of uniformity of impression material within the tray	All areas of the mouth	Complicated fixed procedures

IMPRESSION MATERIAL

Popular impression materials fall into one of two categories of elastomeric materials: polyether (PE) or polyvinyl siloxane (PVS). PE is an elastomeric impression material made of ethylene oxide and tetra-hydrofluro copolymers that polymerize under the effects of an aromatic ester. PVS is an addition reaction of silicone polymer terminal vinyl groups cross linking with silanes under the influence of a platinum or palladium salt catalysis. Both materials enjoy popularity, as they are easy to use and accurate, and possess good technical properties. However, PVS and PE differ in their abilities to wet an intraoral surface and in their wet-ability by dental gypsum materials(3). PE is a hydrophilic material, meaning that it will absorb moisture from its surroundings. PVS is hydrophobic, meaning that it will not take on moisture from its environment. Clinicians are often confused about this fact, believing the opposite is true because it seems that PVS product usage is friendlier in a moist environment than PE.

The property of wet-ability or surface contact angle degree is the property that is manipulated by the manufacturer by the addition of surfactants to alter the true chemical nature of these products. (Contact angle degree = the ability of the impression material to wet the objects being impressed. The lower the contact angle, the greater the wet-ability of the material.)

The properties of rigidity and dimensional stability over time also differ between these two materials. PE is a stiffer material. This is a desirable attribute in implant dentistry, when the impression coping components must be disassembled from the mouth and reassembled in the impression with the laboratory analogs. The confidence that the components are in their correct positions is higher with PE than with the more elastic and flexible PVS(4).

The rigidity of PE is a deterrent in patient comfort and retrieval of the impression. Areas of undercuts or long, periodontally weakened teeth with large interdental spaces will make the removal of this type of impression more difficult. PVS has greater dimensional stability over time than PE but is more sensitive to manipulation variables than PE (5). Movement of the tray once it has been placed will lead to distortion with PVS. Improper injection of the light viscosity material will promote voids. In addition, poor timing of the set of materials of different viscosities will lead to delamination. Failure to use the correct adhesive medium on the tray and/or not allowing it to dry will lead to distortions with both materials.

Latex and hemostatic medicaments are reported to affect impression materials. It is believed the sulfur compounds in the latex gloves inhibit polymerization of PVS. The residue from provisional restorative materials adversely affects the set of PVS (6; see also Table 5.8).

Table 5.8. Impression material selection.

Material	Advantage	Disadvantage	Indications	Contraindications
PVS	Excellent dimensional stability Less ridge than PE Good tear strength Hydrophobic, pleasant taste	Setting inhibition with contact upon latex Sensitive to manipulation variables Delamination of surfaces if contaminated or due to delay in impression placement	All crown and bridge therapy Open tray implant impression procedures	Patients allergic to components
PE	Rigid Dimensionally stable Hydrophilic material Unpleasant taste	Cannot be stored in a moist environment or in contact with wet material Low tear strength	All crown and bridge therapy and open Closed tray implant impression procedures	Patients allergic to components Areas of deep undercut Periodontal weak teeth with large embrasure areas

TISSUE MANAGEMENT

Tissue management is extremely important in the impression-taking process. Countless materials, instruments, medicaments, and techniques have evolved to facilitate the management of gingival tissues for the making of an accurate impression. Retraction cords of various sizes, materials, and fabrication provide mechanical displacement of tissues and enable impression material to enter the submarginal area. Knitted, braided, or twisted cords are the major choices in displacement cord. The purpose is the same in all retraction-cord techniques: the physical displacement of soft tissues by affecting the elastic collagen fibers, altering circumferential periodontal fibers, and controlling sulcular fluids.

Because tissue retraction is a time-consuming procedure, other methods and materials have come into the marketplace in an effort to make this procedure easier and more efficient. Foam displacement materials and hemostatic claylike materials can be used in place of cord to attain displacement of the soft tissues. Electrosurgery and Laser technology offer another approach to soft-tissue displacement. However, one must be cautious in the periodontally challenged patient so as to not create more attachment loss by injudicious application of these technologies. The goal of the process is to acquire an accurate rendition of the submarginal and supramarginal anatomy so that an accurate restoration can be fabricated (Figs. 5.25–5.28).

TECHNOLOGY IN IMPRESSION MAKING

The use of CAD/CAM technology in the making of a digital impression has the potential to irreversibly alter the field of impression taking. ESPE 3M has developed a chairside oral scanner that allows 3D video imaging to be used to capture the prepared teeth. Data are electronically transmitted to the dental laboratory for the fabrication of the dental model and final restoration. The finished restoration is returned for delivery. Cadent iTero has similar optical-scanning hardware and software. The resulting restoration is derived from a model fabricated digitally and sent to the laboratory for final restoration fabrication (Fig. 5.29).

CEREC and E4D have the capacity to provide restorations from virtual models, allowing the dentist to deliver the finished restoration shortly

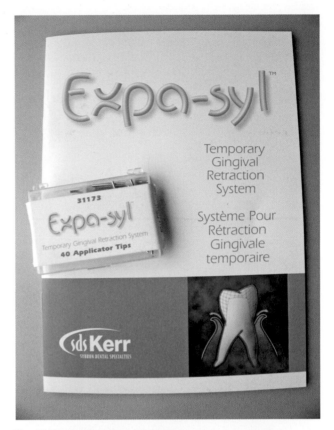

Fig. 5.25 A retraction material.

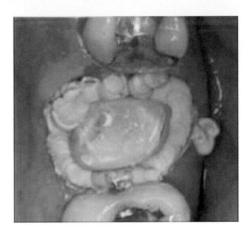

Fig. 5.26 Expa-syl–retraction media is in place.

after the tooth has been prepared and scanned. The milling unit is connected to the scanning unit. The restoration is produced in the dental office by the milling unit.

This technology has been proven to be accurate and successful. It is gaining popularity and will be a major source of indirect restorations in the future as cost and time are reduced for both the dentist and patient.

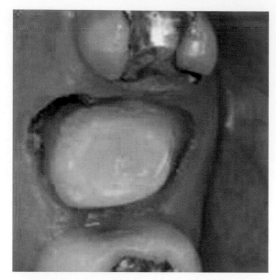

Fig. 5.27 Tissue retraction has been accomplished.

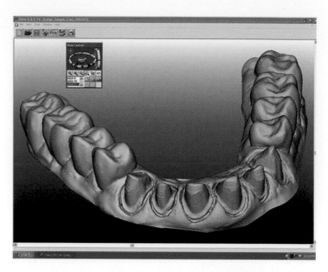

Fig. 5.29 A view of an iTero optical impression.

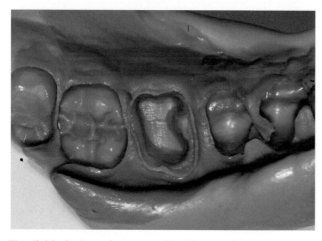

Fig. 5.28 A view of a proper final impression.

References

1. Black GV. Extracts from the Last Century. Susceptibility and Immunity by Dental Caries. BR Dent J 1981;150:10.
2. Rosenstiel SF, Land MF, Fujimoto T. Contemporary fixed prosthodontics 4th ed. St. Louis, Mosby 2006. p. 223.
3. Chee WW, Donovan TE. Polyvinyl siloxane impression materials: A review of properties and techniques. J Prosthetic Dent 1992;68:728–32.
4. Wassell RW, Ibbetson RJ. The accuracy of polyvinyl siloxane impressions made with standard and reinforced stock trays. J Prosthetic Den. 1991;65:748–57.
5. Thongthammachat S, Moore BK, Barco MT, Hovijitra S, Brown DT, Andres CJ. Dimensional accuracy of dental casts: Influence of tray material, impression material, and time. J Prosthodont 2002;11:98–108.
6. De Camargo LM, Chee WW, Donovan TE. Inhibition of polymerization of polyvinyl siloxanes by medicaments used on gingival retraction cords; J Prosthet Dent 1993;70:114–17.

Chapter 6
Developing Treatment Algorithms for Restoration or Replacement of the Compromised Tooth

Paul Fugazzotto and Frederick Hains

The introduction of newer therapeutic modalities, surgical and restorative techniques, and restorative materials has dramatically expanded available treatment options. While a potential boon for clinicians and patients alike, such expansion places greater demands upon the diagnostic and treatment planning capabilities of the clinician. The challenge is not in mastering available surgical and restorative treatment techniques, but rather in determining when to apply each treatment modality, and how to utilize the chosen therapeutic approach to its maximum benefit for the patient.

Treatment decisions should always be made in consideration of the health of the patient, the appropriateness of the therapy, the informed desires of the patient, and the costs of the therapy. Therapeutic costs to be assessed are not only financial, but also biologic, aesthetic, therapeutic, temporal, and psychological. In addition, the prognosis of each therapeutic option over time must be considered.

When faced with a single compromised tooth, treatment options include restoration of the tooth—in conjunction with endodontic, orthodontic, and/or periodontal therapies where necessary—tooth removal and replacement with an implant supported single crown, or tooth removal and replacement with a three-unit fixed partial denture. It is imperative that selection of a specific treatment approach not be grounded in the clinician's less-than-thorough understanding of the advantages, disadvantages, and potentials of each treatment option.

A clinician's lack of understanding or experience with a given treatment approach, or failure to master delivery of such therapy, is a poor excuse for selecting one therapeutic option over another. Rather, treatment outcome expectations, the various risks of each therapeutic option, and the prognosis of each treatment approach should be carefully considered and weighed in the decision-making process.

The challenge is how best to quantify the survival rates of recommended procedures and therapies. While excellent documentation is present regarding success and failure rates of specific therapies, the literature is woefully inadequate in assessing treatment outcomes for other modalities. Many articles poorly define patient selection, the overall patient dental health, criteria for success, and other confounding factors. In addition, a number of published reports utilize materials that are no longer employed on a day-to-day basis. Finally, there is a paucity of literature comparing various treatment approaches in the same patients or clinical practices. As a result, while the goal is to render the decision-making process as scientific as possible, a number of "soft" factors influence this process, including clinician bias and perspective. It is for this reason that clinical dentistry is still a unique combination of art and science.

Diagnostic Requirements

Thorough examination and diagnosis must always be carried out and a comprehensive interdisciplinary treatment plan must be formulated prior to initiation of any active therapy, as discussed in Chapter 1. The components of such an examination will not be repeated here. There are, however, key points that bear mentioning. A thorough examination always begins with an open discussion with the patient, so that the patient's needs and desires may be determined. Failure to ensure such open avenues of communication increases the risk of patient dissatisfaction, and poor treatment outcomes. Thorough data collection is a must. Examination of hard and soft tissues, models with face-bow mountings, and analysis of the patient's occlusion in conjunction with a high-quality full series of radiographs provide base line data needed for decision making and treatment recommendations. Three-dimensional imaging is often required. Such imaging provides especially important information when assessing the bone support on the palatal root of a maxillary molar, the precise extent of an endodontic lesion that is present, the assessment of available bone if tooth extraction and implant placement are contemplated, and assurance of the absence of other pathologies which may either influence the course of therapy or pose significant health risks to the patient.

All potential etiologies must be identified and assessed prior to formulating a comprehensive treatment plan, including systemic factors, periodontal status, the presence or absence of parafunction, carious lesions, endodontic lesions, and trauma.

As the available treatment options and ideal treatment plan are being formulated for presentation to the patient, it is important that both the predictability and expected treatment outcome of each therapeutic approach be honestly and openly assessed and discussed. Such an assessment allows the patient to choose the treatment option for which he or she is best suited physically, financially, and psychologically.

Teeth that can be predictably restored to health through reasonable means should always be maintained, if such retention is advantageous to the final treatment plan and addresses the patient's desires and wishes. Once again, lack of understanding about the predictably attainable results following periodontal and/or endodontic therapy, and the expected long-term prognoses of various approaches, often results in formulation of treatment plans that do a disservice to the patient.

It is inappropriate to remove all teeth that show any degree of compromise and replace them with implant-supported prosthetics. However, it is equally inexcusable to fail to understand and incorporate regenerative and implant therapies into available treatment armentaria, when addressing a patient's unique situation.

The success rates of procedures that have statistical track records can be presented to patients to help them weigh the pros and cons of each therapeutic option. Such data can also be used to support the treatment decisions of the dentist. Unfortunately, the success rate of a particular procedure performed by the practitioner in question, which is of greatest value, is often unavailable statistically. Usually, the dentist can only state that his/her success with this particular procedure is based on the number of times it has been performed successfully. This history of success and/or failure often shapes the treatment plan.

Assessing the Individual Tooth

Prior to making a determination as to the advantages or disadvantages of retaining a given tooth, a number of parameters must be appropriately assessed. Some of these considerations have been discussed in previous chapters and will be briefly reviewed below. A number of salient points to consider include:

The periodontal status of the tooth in question is an absolute indication or contraindication to attempts at long-term maintenance through periodontal and restorative therapies. There is no question that pocket depths in excess of 4mm are not maintainable by either the patient or the dental professional. Therefore, except in instances where teeth are being maintained in older or medically compromised patients, pocket elimination must be a feasible treatment outcome in order to consider restoration and retention of a given tooth. Such pocket elimination may proceed through periodontal resective therapy, periodontal regenerative therapy, or a combination of the two.

Pocket elimination also includes resolution of any furcation involvements that are present. Performing extensive restorative therapy on a furcated tooth because it demonstrates *only* a Class I furcation involvement is ill advised. It is well established that such areas will continue to break down, due to the cul de sac which will continue to trap plaque despite the best professional and patient plaque-control measures. There is no argument in the literature over whether or not furcation involvements progress. The only points to be considered are how quickly a given furcation involvement will progress, the impact of such progression upon the planned therapy, and the influence of overriding patient concerns (age, health, etc.).

As discussed in Chapter 4, a stable band of attached keratinized tissue, and hence an intact fiber barrier system, must be present to help provide adequate defense against the added plaque accumulation and potential periodontal compromise inherent in placement of restorative margins at the gingival crest or intrasulcularly. If such a band of attached keratinized tissue cannot be established due to various anatomic or patient psychological considerations, then the tooth is ill suited for restoration and retention.

The Ability to Safely Perform Crown-Lengthening Surgery

The extent of periodontal attachment loss around the tooth in question, and the expected level of periodontal attachment after necessary periodontal therapy is performed, must be assessed. If a stable periodontal milieu may be established for reception of restorative dentistry without unduly compromising the support of the tooth in question, the argument for retaining the tooth is greatly enhanced. However, should the tooth in question demonstrate extensive periodontal attachment loss, or should performance of necessary preprosthetic crown-lengthening osseous surgery significantly alter the crown-to-root ratio of the tooth, the tooth may be a poor candidate for retention.

A minimum of 3–4 mm of healthy tooth structure must be available crestal to the alveolar bone crest to allow both redevelopment of an appropriate attachment apparatus and establishment of the necessary ferrule in the preparation design. If the restorative margin tooth interface is deep subgingival, patient home care is compromised. The resultant increased plaque accumulation may reinitiate not only the periodontal inflammatory process, but also recurrent caries at the aforementioned interface.

Endodontic Considerations

In addition to determining whether or not endodontic therapy can be carried out on a given tooth, care must be taken to assess the expected residual tooth structure following such endodontic intervention, and the ability of this residual tooth structure to withstand load application over time.

Natural tooth contours may result in a thin isthmus of tooth structure following endodontic therapy. Areas of specific concern are two-rooted maxillary first bicuspids, and the furcal aspect of the mesial root of a lower molar. A study reported from the University of Oregon Dental School found that the teeth with the highest endodontic failure rates were mandibular first premolars, followed by maxillary laterals, maxillary first and second premolars, the mandibular second premolar, and maxillary first molars (1).

While root canal systems are generally predictable in morphology, complicating or unique attributes set many teeth apart. Zillich and Dawson (2) describe mandibular first premolars as either easy or exceedingly difficult to treat. This particular tooth will present with a second or third canal 23% of the time. In addition, these canals may divide at any point within the root. Maxillary premolars exhibit variations similar to mandibular premolars, often making them difficult to successfully treat.

Sjogren et al. report 8–10-year success rates of 96% in teeth with vital pulps and 86% if the pulp was necrotic, following endodontic therapy (3). The manner in which the tooth is obturated affects success. However, endodontic success does not always equate to restorative success. The factors confounding endodontic therapy make restorative options more challenging. Placement of a post in a maxillary or mandibular first premolar that falls in the 23% complex root canal configuration category may be impossible or result in a compromised prognosis, due to the mechanics of preparing the internal aspect of an irregular cavity with walls of varying thickness using a rotary instrument. The absolute and relative contraindications to retention of a given tooth are listed in Table 6.1.

Periodontal stability, defined as no probing depths greater than 3 mm and no horizontal furcation involvements, must be attainable so as to provide a milieu that is accessible to the patient for effective home-care measures. The inability to do so is an absolute contraindication to tooth retention.

The inability to perform the necessary endodontic therapy on the tooth in question must also

Table 6.1. Relative fees for various therapies.

Therapy	Fee
Endodontics—Single root	0.9X
Endodontics—Multiple root	1.3X
Core buildup—Natural tooth	0.6X
Crown—Natural tooth	1.3X
Pontic	1.4X
Crown-lengthening periodontal surgery	1.1X
Regenerative periodontal surgery	1.9X
Orthodontic supereruption	2.8X
Extraction	0.3X
Three-unit fixed bridge	4.3X
Implant	2.1X
Implant abutment (stock) and crown	2.2X
Implant abutment (custom) and crown	2.7X
Regenerative therapy at tooth extraction	0.7–1.4X
Sinus augmentation	2.5X
Osteotome sinus lift	0.9X
Osteotome sinus lift at time of implant placement	N/C

be seen as an absolute contraindication to tooth retention.

If tooth extraction and implant placement are to be contemplated, it is important to realize that such a treatment choice does not preclude the need for appropriate diagnosis and assessment before carrying out therapy.

Implant Receptor Site Considerations

The implant option is not without its own set of conditions, which need to be evaluated.

A number of site-specific factors must be considered if tooth removal and implant placement are to be entertained. The position of the implant recipient bone is of paramount importance, as are the quantity and quality of the available bone. A malpositioned tooth may result in an extraction socket whose position precludes ideal implant positioning without either regenerative therapy at the time of tooth extraction followed by subsequent implant placement, or concomitant regenerative therapy at the time of tooth removal and implant insertion.

It is crucial that the assessment of bone quantity be carried out in a three-dimensional manner. All too often, such an assessment is limited to evaluating the length of the implant that may be placed, and whether or not the implant will be inserted wholly within an intact extraction socket. Such an assessment is inadequate. A patient with a thin, highly scalloped biotype or one who has undergone buccal orthodontic tooth movement, or has caused hard- and soft-tissue recession through aggressive brushing, will demonstrate a thin, highly labile buccal alveolar bony plate following tooth removal. Placement of an implant in such a situation without concomitant regenerative therapy to protect and increase the bulk of the buccal bone will leave the patient with a situation highly prone to either postoperative bone resorption, or bone resorption upon application of functional load. Any implant placed must be housed in adequate bone to withstand functional forces buccally and lingually/palatally, over time.

Assessing Cost-Benefit Ratios

In dentistry, extrapolation is made from the combined experience of treating many patients and evidence from literature when making treatment decisions. However, it is important to realize that humans are unique, and one case may not have the same outcome as others treated in the same manner. A risk-reward benefits analysis must be undertaken to help determine the most reasonable approach to a given situation. The development of an appropriate treatment algorithm mandates recognition and evaluation of all applicable cost-benefit ratios. These cost-benefit ratios are biologic, esthetic, financial, temporal, psychological and therapeutic in nature. Appropriate assessment must also take into consideration not only the present, but also the future status of the treatment delivered.

BIOLOGIC CONSIDERATIONS

Biologic costs impact both the tooth under direct consideration and adjacent teeth. The tooth being assessed may pay a biologic price in terms of loss of tooth structure following preparation with or without endodontic intervention, loss of supporting bone following preprosthetic periodontal therapy when necessary, or development of furcation involvements following preprosthetic crown-lengthening osseous surgery.

CLINICAL EXAMPLE ONE

A patient presents with a subgingival fracture on the buccal aspect of a mandibular first molar (Fig. 6.1). This tooth has already undergone endodontic therapy. Radiographic examination (Fig. 6.2) dem-

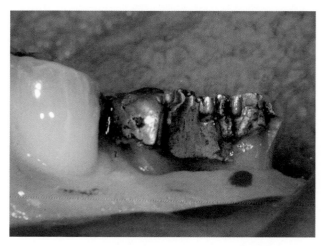

Fig. 6.1 A patient presents with a buccal subgingival fracture of a mandibular first molar.

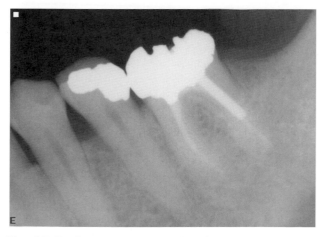

Fig. 6.2 Radiographic examination demonstrates a short residual root trunk between the fracture and the entrance to the buccal furcation. Performance of crown-lengthening osseous surgery would result in a significant buccal furcation involvement on the first molar.

onstrates the short residual root trunk which is present between the root fracture and the entrance to the buccal furcation. Due to the short distance between the subgingival margin of the buccal fracture and the entrance to the furcation (approximately 1.3 mm), performance of the necessary crown-lengthening osseous surgery would result in development of a significant buccal furcation involvement, and a compromised prognosis for the tooth following completion of therapy.

Removal of such a tooth and its replacement by an implant with concomitant regenerative therapy may appear at first to be an overly aggressive treatment approach. The argument might be made that the patient would be better served by placing a crown on the tooth and "trying to hold on to it for as long as possible," especially as endodontic therapy had been performed some years before. However, such a treatment option is not in the best interest of the patient unless patient health precludes more comprehensive care, or patient age leads the clinician to believe that the tooth will not have to function for much longer.

Post and core build-buildup and a full coverage restoration without periodontal surgical therapy entails significant expense, and will result in a milieu that institutes a periodontal inflammatory lesion almost immediately upon completion of tooth restoration. At best, the disease process will proceed slowly. At worst, the tooth will become significantly compromised and periodontally untreatable in the near future.

Performance of crown-lengthening osseous surgery prior to post and core buildup and full-coverage restoration of the tooth will entail additional expense, and will not provide a periodontal milieu conducive to placement of restorative dentistry without the initiation of an inflammatory periodontal lesion. Conservative therapy is removal of the tooth, placement of an implant, and subsequent restoration so as to provide a healthy, functional situation for the patient.

The biologic costs to the adjacent teeth must also be considered. If crown-lengthening osseous surgery performed around a given tooth will unduly compromise the periodontal support of the adjacent teeth, such therapy is not indicated. It is hard to justify performing treatment that compromises healthy teeth, when predictable therapeutic modalities such as tooth extraction and implant placement exist. Fig. 6.3 demonstrates a mandibular first molar with recurrent subgingival caries on its distal aspect. The position of the caries is such that

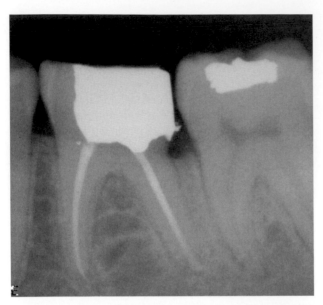

Fig. 6.3 A patient presents with recurrent subgingival caries on the distal aspect of the mandibular first molar. The position of the caries renders this tooth an excellent candidate for crown-lengthening osseous surgery.

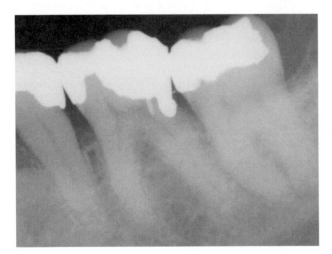

Fig. 6.4 A patient presents with recurrent subgingival caries on the distal aspect of the mandibular first molar. Crown-lengthening osseous surgery would necessitate removal of significant bone support from the mesial aspect of the mandibular second molar, and may compromise the entrance to the buccal furcation of the mandibular first molar. The first molar should be removed and replaced.

crown-lengthening osseous surgery can be safely performed without unduly compromising the supporting bone of either the first molar or the mesial aspect of the second molar. In contrast, Fig. 6.4 is

a radiograph of a mandibular first molar, which demonstrates recurrent subgingival caries on its distal aspect that represents a much greater compromise than that encountered in Fig. 6.3. Due to the extension of the caries along the distal root, appropriate crown-lengthening osseous surgery would involve removal of significant osseous support and attachment apparatus from the mesial aspect of the second molar, as well as a possible inability to attain the necessary biologic width between the recurrent caries and the entrance to the buccal furcation of the first molar. It is important to remember that 4 mm of exposed tooth structure must be available for restoration in all directions from carious lesions.

CLINICAL EXAMPLE TWO

A patient presents with recurrent caries around a crown on a maxillary second bicuspid (Fig. 6.5). This caries is on the distal surface of the second bicuspid. If the caries had been located on the buccal or palatal aspects of the tooth, crown-lengthening osseous surgery could safely be performed without affecting the support of the adjacent teeth. However, because the subgingival caries was on the distal aspect of the second bicuspid, performance of the necessary crown-lengthening osseous surgery would significantly compromise the mesial support, and result in development of a mesial furcation involvement, of the adjacent first

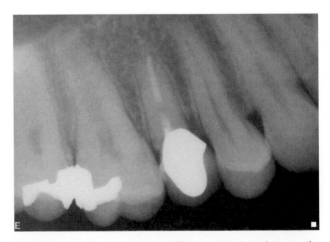

Fig. 6.5 A patient presents with recurrent caries on the distal aspect of the second premolar. Crown-lengthening osseous surgery would result in significant compromise of the bone support on the mesial aspect of the second molar, and invasion of the mesial furcation of the second molar.

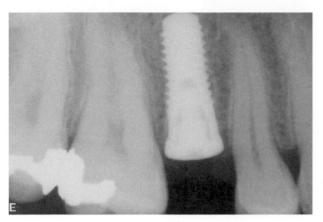

Fig. 6.6 The tooth is removed and replaced with an implant.

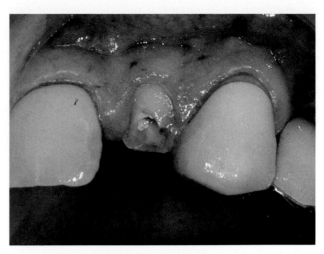

Fig. 6.7 Crown-lengthening osseous surgery on the fractured maxillary lateral incisor would yield an unsatisfactory aesthetic result unless supereruption were first performed. Utilization of supereruption followed by crown-lengthening surgery in such a situation would result in a poor crown-to-root ratio following tooth restoration.

molar. As a result, it was more prudent to remove the tooth and place an implant at the time of tooth removal (Fig. 6.6).

AESTHETIC CONSIDERATIONS

The effects of crown-lengthening osseous surgery on the patient's aesthetics must be assessed. While palatal caries on a maxillary anterior tooth may be safely exposed for restoration, the same procedure performed interproximally or buccally often results in an unacceptable aesthetic treatment outcome. In such situations, other treatment options should be explored. Fig. 6.7 demonstrates such a situation. If crown-lengthening osseous surgery were performed around the subgingivally fractured lateral incisor, the final treatment result would represent a significant aesthetic compromise. If the maxillary lateral incisor is to be maintained, it must be supererupted prior to crown-lengthening osseous surgery. As already discussed, such an approach is not ideal, as the supererupted, crown-lengthened, and restored lateral incisor would present with a poor crown-root ratio and thus a limited prognosis, after the patient had been subjected to extensive and expensive therapies.

FINANCIAL CONSIDERATIONS

The financial ramifications of each treatment approach play a significant role in selection of a given therapeutic modality. In order to better assess this consideration, a questionnaire was sent to 100 periodontists in urban and suburban areas throughout the United States. The periodontists were asked, in consultation with their restorative partners, to provide information regarding the costs of various therapies. Eighty-seven periodontists sent back the requested information. As a result, 13 additional periodontists were individually contacted, and asked to provide the same information. Each of them did so, affording a database of 100 periodontists and their restorative partners throughout the United States. The cost data from this survey are documented in Table 6.1. The average cost of restoration of a natural tooth was 1.3X. If crown-lengthening osseous surgery was required, an additional cost of 1.1X was added for a total cost of 2.4X. Should endodontic therapy be necessary, an additional fee of 0.9X–1.3X was added, for a total fee of 3.3X–3.7X. Finally, if a core buildup was carried out after endodontic therapy, an additional 0.6X of cost was added for a total fee of 3.9X to 4.3X.

The average cost of tooth extraction, implant placement, and restoration with a stock abutment and single crown was 4.6X. If regenerative therapy was necessary in conjunction with implant placement, an additional fee of 0.7X–1.4X was added for a total fee of 5.3X–6.0X.

Considering only the financial ramifications of therapy, it becomes obvious that, if a tooth may be restored in a healthy manner necessitating either crown-lengthening osseous surgery or endodontic therapy and post and core buildup, it is prudent to do so. However, if crown-lengthening periodontal surgery, endodontic therapy, post and core buildup, and full-coverage restoration are required on a given tooth, and the tooth could instead be replaced with an implant, abutment, and crown without performing extensive regenerative therapy, it is more logical financially to follow the implant course of treatment. Naturally, financial considerations do not stand alone in determining the appropriate therapeutic approach.

TEMPORAL CONSIDERATIONS

Temporal requirements must also be considered. If tooth retention mandates an excessive number of visits to perform the necessary periodontal therapy, endodontic therapy, and subsequent restoration, the patient may be better served through tooth extraction and implant placement at the time of tooth removal. Following healing, two restorative visits will usually be required. However, implant reconstructive therapy will be viewed in such a manner only if all treating clinicians understand the potentials of various therapeutic approaches.

The ability to extract a tooth, debride the socket, and successfully place an implant at the time of tooth removal, with or without immediate temporization, has been well established throughout the literature. Numerous articles have elucidated various treatment algorithms for implant placement at the time of tooth removal (4). The literature conclusively demonstrates that the predictability of osseointegration if implants are placed at the time of tooth extraction, or are placed into intact bone following healing, is essentially the same when considering implant placement at the time of extraction of single-rooted teeth.

Implant placement at the time of multirooted tooth extraction has traditionally been viewed as a compromised treatment approach due to the technical difficulties in ideally positioning the implant, and the unpredictability in effecting appropriate regeneration of bone in the residual extraction socket surrounding the implant. However, two recent publications documenting over 650 cases demonstrate the long-term predictability of implant placement at the time of extraction of maxillary or mandibular molars, with performance of concomitant regenerative therapy (5, 6).

Immediate implant placement at the time of tooth extraction should not be viewed as a compromise, but rather as another therapeutic alternative to be considered when developing viable treatment algorithms. Immediate implant placement at the time of tooth extraction may also shorten the time required to perform therapy. Utilization of such a treatment approach will often result in a significantly shorter course of therapy than crown-lengthening osseous therapy, endodontic therapy after appropriate healing has occurred, and post and core buildup and restoration of the tooth in question.

PSYCHOLOGICAL CONSIDERATIONS

Patient demands and desires may lead to selection of one treatment approach over the other. If a patient is psychologically unable to deal with the thought of losing his or her tooth, or is afraid of having an implant placed, extraordinary efforts may be made in attempting to save the tooth in question. Patient desires may also mandate tooth extraction and replacement with an implant. A patient who is ill suited for complex multidisciplinary care, or one who states that he or she does not wish to maintain a given tooth and subject it to extensive therapy "unless the result is guaranteed," is a poor candidate for performance of crown-lengthening osseous surgery, endodontic therapy, and tooth restoration.

Complexity of Care

Complexity of care is an important consideration. A tooth for which performance of appropriate endodontic therapy would be difficult if not impossible is ill suited for retention. In addition, if the complexity of surgical and/or restorative therapy required increases the chances of immediate or long-term failure, tooth retention is not advised.

Implant utilization does not eliminate all concerns regarding complexity of care and the required clinical skills to perform appropriate therapy. Surgical access, site compromises, or difficulty in restoration following osseointegration of the implant are all serious contraindications to tooth removal and implant placement.

Predictability of Care

The long-term predictability of therapy is paramount when selecting a treatment approach. There is a paucity of literature comparing long-term success rates of teeth restored with single crowns, with or without prior endodontic intervention, and single-implant-supported crowns. A comparison of studies purporting to evaluate one or the other of the treatment modalities is difficult. Significant advances in endodontic techniques and restorative materials render many of the older studies of no use in carrying out such a comparison. In addition, the advent of rough-surfaced implants and various implant designs and restorative options invalidates the inclusion of older studies when comparing long-term success rates of different treatment approaches. Available literature assessing success rates of teeth restored with single crowns, with or without prior endodontic therapy and utilizing newer restorative materials, reports success rates in the range of 94% (7). Implant success and survival rates for rough-surface implants restored with single crowns have been consistently reported in excess of 95% over 5 to 10 years (8).

Prior to the advent of implant therapy, steps were taken to retain as many "pieces" of multi-rooted teeth as possible to help support fixed reconstructive therapy.

CLINICAL EXAMPLE THREE

A patient presented 28 years ago with a limited number of retained maxillary and mandibular teeth, and significant periodontal disease around all teeth that did remain. Following placement of full-arch maxillary and mandibular temporary fixed splints, the maxillary left first molar and second bicuspid were treated periodontally. Flap reflection demonstrated severe osseous loss, and a significant buccal furcation involvement on the maxillary first molar (Fig. 6.8). An occlusal view also demonstrated a deep distal furcation involvement on the first molar (Fig. 6.9). Fortunately, the mesial furcation of the tooth was intact. As a result of these findings, the tooth was sectioned and the distobuccal root was removed. Fig. 6.10 demonstrates the excellent intrafurcal bone remaining between the two residual roots of the first molar. Appropriate osseous therapy and odontoplasty were carried out. The odontoplasty served both to

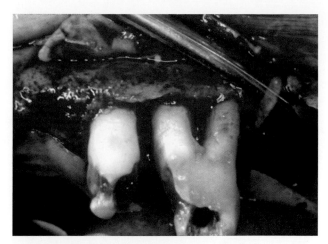

Fig. 6.8 Flap reflection demonstrates a deep buccal furcation involvement on the maxillary first molar.

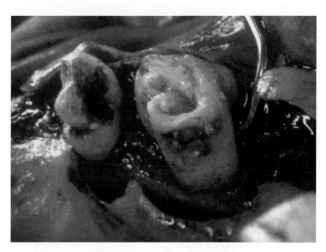

Fig. 6.9 An occlusal view demonstrates a deep distal furcation involvement on the maxillary first molar.

eliminate a Class I mesial furcation involvement on the first molar, and to ensure that the emergence profile of the residual tooth out of the bone was straight (Fig. 6.11). Following crestal anticipation of the palatal flap, the buccal and palatal muco-periosteal flaps were sutured at osseous crest utilizing interrupted 4-0 silk sutures (Fig. 6.12). Once healing was complete, modification of the maxillary provisional restoration was carried out. The emergence profile out of the gingiva in the area of root resection was straight. The contours of the provisional restoration then flowed into the desired occlusal contours (Fig. 6.13). Although no opposing tooth was present in the area of the first molar,

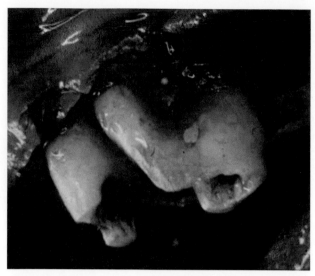

Fig. 6.10 Following tooth sectioning and removal of the distobuccal root of the maxillary first molar, the furcation between the mesiobuccal and palatal roots demonstrates an intact attachment apparatus and excellent alveolar bone support.

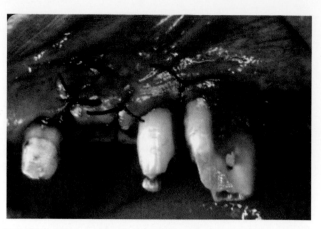

Fig. 6.12 The mucoperiosteal flaps are sutured at osseous crest with interrupted 4-0 silk sutures.

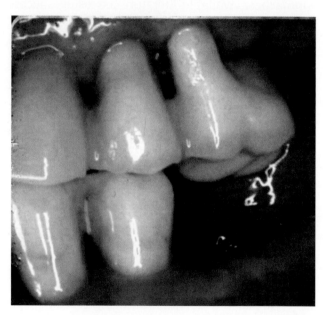

Fig. 6.13 A provisional restoration has been placed following appropriate healing. Note the straight emergence profile of the provisional restoration out of the gingiva in the area of root resection.

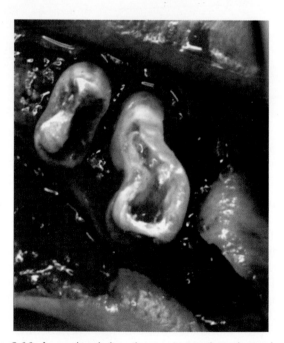

Fig. 6.11 An occlusal view demonstrates the odontoplasty that has been performed on the maxillary first molar to eliminate a Class I mesial furcation involvement and to ensure that the emergence profile of the tooth out of the bone is straight in the area of root resection.

the maxillary first molar was retained to help add support to the planned full arch fixed splint.

The incorporation of implant therapy into overall patient care significantly aids the clinician in avoiding such complex and demanding therapies. By placing implants in key locations, additional abutments may be provided, and a simpler reconstructive effort may be undertaken.

CLINICAL EXAMPLE FOUR

Root resective therapy, in conjunction with crown-lengthening osseous surgery, can afford the patient a high degree of predictability when utilized in appropriate situations. A patient presents with periodontal pocketing around all teeth in the maxillary left quadrant, a deep Class II buccal to distal furcation involvement on the maxillary first molar, and inadequate clinical tooth structure for appropriate restoration (Fig. 6.14). The concave, inflamed interproximal col forms between the teeth are evident clinically (Fig. 6.15). A Class I buccal furcation involvement is evident on the maxillary first molar (Fig. 6.16). An occlusal view (Fig. 6.17) demonstrates the odontoplasty that was carried out in an effort to eliminate the buccal furcation

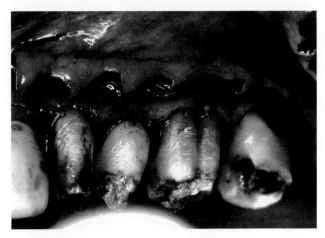

Fig. 6.16 Flap reflection demonstrates a Class II buccal furcation involvement on the maxillary first molar.

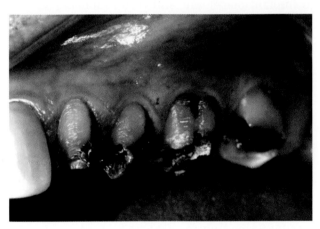

Fig. 6.14 A patient presents with inadequate clinical crown length for appropriate tooth restoration, and a deep Class II buccal furcation involvement on the maxillary first molar.

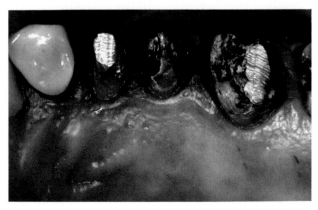

Fig. 6.15 An occlusal view demonstrates the concave, inflamed nature of the soft-tissue cols between the teeth.

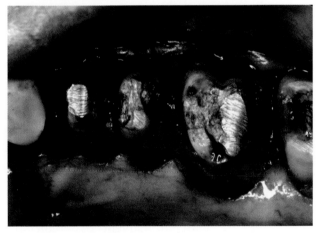

Fig. 6.17 An occlusal view highlights efforts made to eliminate the buccal furcation involvement on the maxillary first molar utilizing odontoplasty. Unfortunately, a significant horizontal component to the furcation involvement remained. Extension of the internal aspect of the furcation involvement between the mesiobuccal and palatal roots of the tooth precluded appropriate debridement to effect regenerative therapy.

involvement on the first molar. Unfortunately, a significant horizontal component to the furcation involvement still remained. In addition, as the internal aspect of the furcation involvement extended between the mesiobuccal and palatal roots of the tooth, this area could not be appropriately debrided to attempt regenerative therapy. As a result, tooth sectioning with removal of the mesiobuccal root was carried out (Fig. 6.18). The

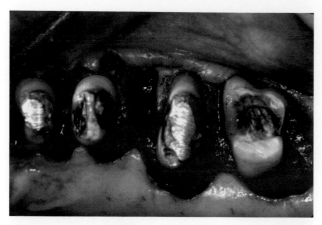

Fig. 6.18 The maxillary first molar is sectioned and the mesiobuccal root is removed. Note the elimination of the Class I furcation involvements on the second molar through the use of odontoplasty.

Class I furcation involvements on the second molar were eliminated through odontoplasty. Appropriate biologic width was attained around all teeth, and osseous resective therapy was performed as necessary to eliminate osseous defects and ensure positive osseous architecture. Following healing, these teeth can be predictably restored with full-coverage restorations, after endodontic therapy has been carried out on the first molar.

While root resective therapy and subsequent restoration are a predictable, proven treatment modality, they must be utilized judiciously. This is especially true with the advent of predictable implant reconstructive treatment modalities. The previous clinical example demonstrates a situation in which retention of the maxillary first molar was highly predictable and obviated the need for implant therapy. However, such a scenario is not always what the treating clinicians face.

The Cost of Retreatment

The commitment necessary upon retreatment must also be carefully weighed. Failure of a natural tooth restored with a single crown may be due to crown fracture, recurrent caries, root fracture, development of an endodontic lesion, or progressive periodontal disease. The dangers of root fractures following endodontic therapy which results in inadequate tooth structure to withstand functional forces over time have already been reviewed. Most of the complications listed above would result in significant retreatment, or tooth removal and replacement.

In contrast, complications around osseointegrated rough-surface implants restored with cemented single crowns usually take the form of porcelain fracture, or soft-tissue inflammation. The inflammation is easily treated through debridement and/or mucogingival therapy. Depending upon the method that had been employed to attach the crown to the implant, treatment may require either removal of the crown and application of new porcelain, or replacement of the crown. Either need is less involved and less traumatic to the patient than tooth removal and replacement. Naturally, a third treatment option is tooth removal and placement of a three-unit fixed partial denture. An in-depth discussion of this option, as compared to implant placement and restoration for replacement of a single missing tooth, has been explored in detail and will not be discussed here (9).

CLINICAL EXAMPLE FIVE

A patient presented with extensive periodontal destruction in the maxillary left posterior sextant. The maxillary first and second premolars were hopeless. A Class III buccal to mesial furcation involvement was noted on the maxillary first molar. The maxillary premolars were extracted and implants were placed with concomitant regenerative therapy. Crown-lengthening osseous surgery was performed on the first and second molars, in conjunction with a mesiobuccal root resection on the maxillary first molar. Examination of the master cast demonstrates implant positions, as well as the contour attained on the maxillary first molar following root resection and appropriate odontoplasty (Fig. 6.19). Castings were fabricated on the implants and natural teeth, ensuring that a straight emergence profile of the casting from the gingival was present in the area of root resection (Fig. 6.20). Five years later, the second molar decayed and had to be removed. At the time of tooth extraction, it was replaced by an implant, which was subsequently restored with a single crown. Six years later, 11 years after the initial surgical therapy was carried out, the patient presented with significant recurrent decay on the retained roots of the maxillary first molar (Figs. 6.21, 6.22). This tooth will now have to be extracted and replaced with an implant. While 5 and 11 years, respectively, fall

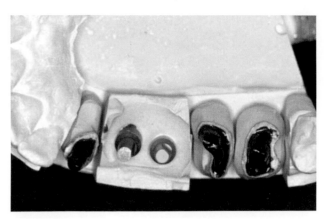

Fig. 6.19 Implants are in place in the positions of the first and second premolars. A mesiobuccal root amputation has been performed on the first molar. Crown-lengthening osseous surgery has been performed on the second molar.

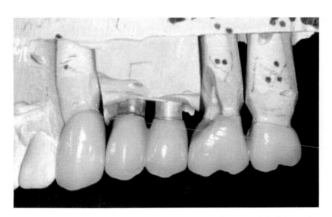

Fig. 6.20 The castings are in place on the model. Note the straight emergence profile of the casting out of the gingiva in the area of the mesiobuccal root amputation on the maxillary first molar.

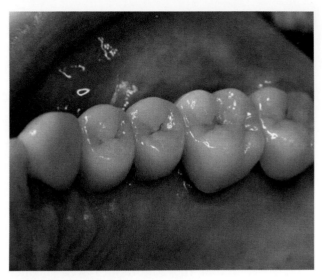

Fig. 6.21 Eleven years postoperatively, the second molar has already been replaced by an abutment and crown. Recurrent caries is now noted around the retained roots of the first molar.

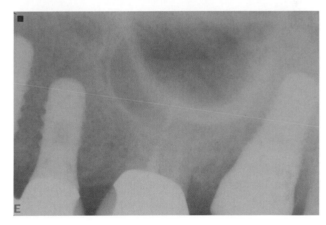

Fig. 6.22 A radiograph demonstrates recurrent caries on the retained roots of the maxillary first molar.

within accepted time frames for assessing treatment success, the patient was not well served by this therapeutic approach. As significant reconstructive and implant therapy was already being carried out, and as the patient demonstrated a relatively high caries rate, it would have been more logical to extract the premolars and molars, place four implants with concomitant regeneration, and restore them with individual abutments and crowns.

The financial costs of multiple procedures performed on a tooth may appear excessive if the prognosis or expected outcome of treatment deteriorates. In addition, each therapy represents an inconvenience to the patient, possible discomfort, and a healing period. Should multiple procedures be chosen to accomplish a goal if an approach requiring fewer visits would afford the same treatment outcome, expectations, and prognosis of the therapy? Training has traditionally advocated preservation of a given tooth as the optimal therapy to offer to a patient. However, hidden unknowns such as an undetected crack in the tooth, damage to the root wall during post preparation, an exposed furcation due to a necessary crown-lengthening procedure, a root system that has unrealized complexities, or an endodontic fill that is "only clinically acceptable," conspire to yield a result whose unpredictable prognosis cannot be calculated.

CLINICAL EXAMPLE SIX

A patient presented in 1981 with recurrent caries around a cantilevered four-unit fixed prosthesis (Fig. 6.23). Following removal of the fixed prosthesis, the subgingival extension of the recurrent carious lesions was evident (Fig. 6.24). Crown-lengthening osseous surgery was carried out, and the buccal and palatal mucoperiosteal flaps were sutured at osseous crest, as previously described (Fig. 6.25). Care was taken to remove as little soft tissue as possible while still attaining the necessary tooth exposure. Following replacement of the fixed splint as a provisional prosthesis, the amount of additional tooth that had been exposed was evident (Fig. 6.26). Examination at a postoperative visit demonstrated that the soft tissues were healing well, at the desired levels (Fig. 6.27).

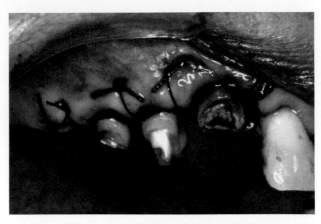

Fig. 6.25 Following appropriate crown-lengthening osseous surgery, the buccal and palatal mucoperiosteal flaps are sutured at osseous crest with interrupted 4-0 silk sutures.

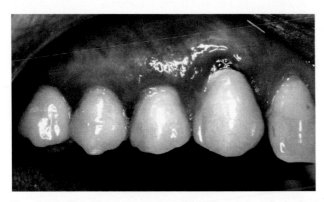

Fig. 6.23 A patient presents with recurrent subgingival caries around the three abutments of a four-unit, cantilevered, fixed prosthesis.

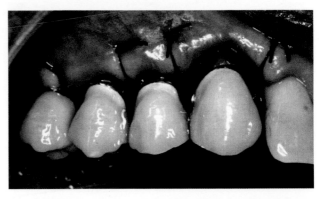

Fig. 6.26 Replacement of the four-unit, fixed prosthesis, which is now being utilized as a provisional restoration, demonstrates the efforts that were made to remove as little soft tissue as possible from the maxillary cuspid, while still attaining the required clinical crown length.

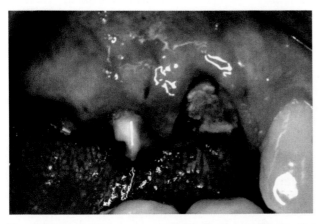

Fig. 6.24 Following removal of the fixed prosthesis, the subgingival extension of the recurrent caries is evident.

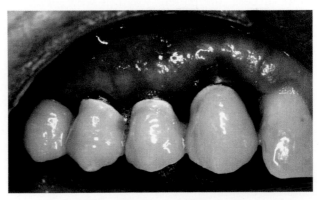

Fig. 6.27 A postoperative view demonstrates healing of the soft tissues at the desired levels.

When the above therapy was carried out in 1981, predictable implant treatment was not an option. As such, crown-lengthening osseous surgery had to be performed, and a new four-unit cantilevered fixed prosthesis was fabricated and inserted. Such a treatment approach would represent a number of compromises today. There is no doubt that a cantilever should not be employed. Rather, a single implant should be placed in the first molar position and restored with an abutment and crown. If necessary, transalveolar augmentation could be carried out prior to or at the time of implant placement. Utilization of a short implant in such a situation results in significantly less force transmission to the bone and the adjacent teeth than fabrication of a cantilevered fixed prosthesis. In addition, if crown-lengthening osseous surgery were to be carried out, orthodontic supereruption would first be performed on the cuspid, so as to extrude hard and soft tissues and afford the opportunity to perform crown-lengthening osseous surgery without negatively impacting the aesthetic treatment outcome. Finally, a decision would have to be made as to whether it was more prudent to maintain the decayed and endodontically treated cuspid and premolars, or to remove them and replace them with implants, abutments. and crowns. In the situation demonstrated in Clinical Example Six, these teeth would be maintained, as the caries had not extended down the roots of the teeth and was easily exposed by crown-lengthening osseous surgery, while leaving more than adequate tooth structure and bone support for the teeth to function successfully over time.

Such is not always the case. If the caries on the teeth has significantly compromised the root surfaces either by extending deep subgingivally, or by resulting in thin residual intact tooth structure which would be prone to fracture after post and core buildup, restoration and force application, tooth removal and implant placement are indicated.

CLINICAL EXAMPLE SEVEN

A patient presents with significant caries on the maxillary first and second premolars and the maxillary second molar (Fig. 6.28). The maxillary first molar is missing. Due to a combination of the extension of caries subgingivally, and caries having destroyed much of the bulk of the tooth mesially and distally, it was more prudent to extract

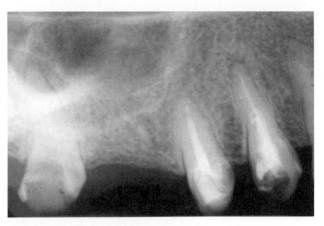

Fig. 6.28 A patient presents with deep, recurrent caries on the maxillary first and second premolars and maxillary second molar.

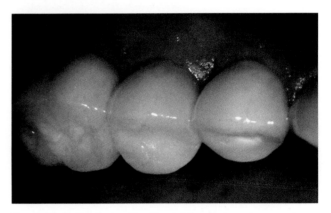

Fig. 6.29 Following extraction of the first and second premolars and second molar, implants were placed and restored in both premolar and the first molar positions.

the three teeth and place implants in the positions of the first and second premolars, and the first molar. No opposing mandibular tooth was present in the second molar position. Subsequent to attainment of osseointegration, the implants were restored with abutments and crowns (Fig. 6.29). Radiographic examination 8 years after therapy demonstrates stability of the peri-implant crestal bone (Fig. 6.30).

Single-tooth replacement with osseointegrated implants and crown restorations has proven to be a highly predictable treatment modality. Numerous longitudinal and retrospective studies demonstrate survival rates at least equal to other methods of tooth replacement, over time (8, 10–12). Jivraj and Chee state, "Decisions to salvage questionable teeth should be weighed against the

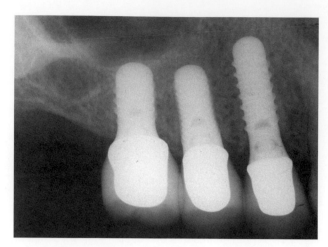

Fig. 6.30 A radiograph taken 8 years post-therapy demonstrates stability of the peri-implant crestal bone.

predictability of implant therapy and the efficacy of long term outcomes."

Does this mean that all decayed teeth, or teeth requiring endodontic therapy, should be extracted and replaced by implants? It does not. Such a treatment approach is unjustifiable. There is no doubt that crown-lengthening therapy, followed by appropriate restorative intervention, is highly predictable. However, such treatment should not be blindly performed without appropriately assessing other available therapeutic modalities (Table 6.2).

Conclusion

A number of treatment options afford themselves to the clinician when faced with a compromised tooth. However, prior to determining which treatment approach to pursue, whether it be tooth retention with periodontal and/or endodontic therapy, or tooth removal, implant placement, and restoration, the indications, contraindications, potentials, and risks of each treatment approach must be assessed (Flow Chart 6.1). The final decision should be based on what is in the best interest of the patient, and not be determined by the clinician's diagnostic or clinical limitations.

References

1. Miller HM. Incidence of extraction at the U of Oregon Dental School. Oral Surg 1958;11: 1226–28.

Table 6.2. Local factors influencing when to perform crown-lengthening osseous surgery (CLS).

Factor	Perform CLS and keep tooth	Remove tooth
Can make tooth periodontally stable[1]	Y	N[2]
Can treat the tooth endodontically	Y	N[2]
Will compromise adjacent support	N	Y[2]
Will induce secondary occlusal trauma	N	Y[3]
Requires periodontal, endodontic, and restorative therapies	N	Y[3]
Presence of parafunction	N	Y[3]
Aesthetic compromise following therapy	N	Y[3]
Large number of visits required	N	Y[3]
Complex therapy required	N	Y[3]
Long-term prognosis excellent	Y	N[2]
Patient wants to keep tooth	Y	N[3]

[1]Denotes probing depths ≤3mm; no furcation involvements; adequate attached keratinized tissue.
[2]Absolute indication for tooth removal.
[3]Relative indication for therapy.

2. Zillich R, Dawson J. Root canal morphology of the mandibular 1st and 2nd premolars. Oral Surg. 1973;36: 738–44.

3. Sjogren U, Hagglund B, Sundqvist G, Wing K. J Endod 1990:10:498–504.

4. Fugazzotto PA. Treatment options following single rooted tooth removal: A literature review and proposed hierarchy of treatment selection. J Periodontol 2005;76: 821–31.

5. Fugazzotto PA. Implant placement at the time of maxillary molar extraction: Treatment options and reported results. J Periodontol, 2008;79:216–23.

6. Fugazzotto PA. Implant placement at the time of mandibular molar extraction: Description of technique

and preliminary results of 341 cases. J Periodontol 2008;79:737–47.

7. Salinas TJ, Eckert SE. In Patients requiring single tooth replacement, what are the outcomes of implants as compared to tooth supported restorations? Int J Oral Maxillofac Implants 2007;22:71–92.

8. Fugazzotto PA, Vlassis J, Butler B. Success and failure rates of 5,526 ITI implants in function for up to 73+ months. Int J Oral Maxillofac Implants 2004;19: 408–12.

9. Fugazzotto PA. Decision making when replacing a missing tooth. Dent Clin N Amer 2009;53: 9–129.

10. Schmitt A, Zarb GA. The longitudinal clinical effectiveness of osseointegrated dental implants for single tooth replacement. Int J Prosthodontic 1993;6: 187–202.

11. Ekfeldt A, Carlsson GE, Borgesson G. Clinical evaluation of single tooth restorations supported by osseointegrated implants: A retrospective study. Int J Oral Maxillofac Implants 1994;9: 179–83.

12. Becker W, Becker BE. Replacement of maxillary and mandibular molars with single endosseous implant restorations: Aa retrospective study. J Prosthet Dent 1995;74: 51–55.

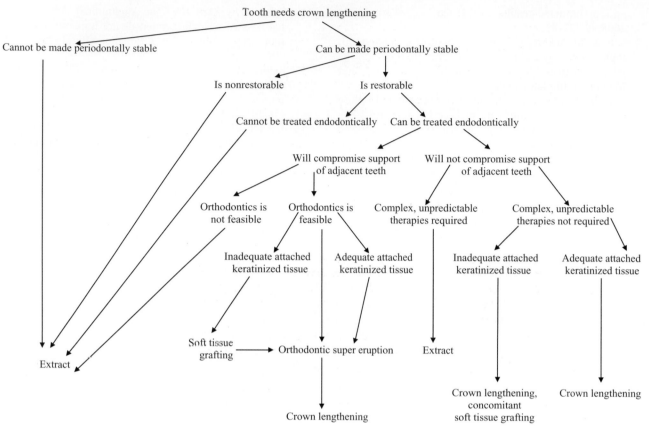

Flow chart 6.1 A tooth requiring crown lengthening.

Index

Note: Italicized page locators indicate a photo/figure; tables are noted with a *t*.